# THE UN–DIET
# BOOK

The all–natural lifestyle for weight loss
and eating, good health and exercise
by the author of THE UNCOOK BOOK

## Elizabeth Baker

D0937612

## DRELWOOD PUBLICATIONS

Distributed by:
DRELWOOD COMMUNICATIONS INC.
P. O. Box 149
Indianola, WA  98342

Although the authors and publisher have exhaustively researched all sources to ensure the accuracy and completeness of the information contained in this book, we assume no responsibility for errors, inaccuracies, omissions or any inconsistency herein. Any slights of people or organizations are unintentional. Readers should use their own judgment, consult a holistic medical expert or their personal physicians for specific applications to their individual problems.

Library of Congress Cataloging in Publication Data

Baker, Elizabeth, 1913-
    Un-Diet Book
    Bibliography: p.
    1.  Food, Natural.   2.  Cookery (Natural foods)
    3.  Health
ISBN 0-937766-17-8

**ATTENTION: SCHOOLS, ORGANIZATIONS AND COMPANIES:** Drelwood Communication Inc. books are availabe at quantity discounts with bulk purchases for educational, business or sales promotional use. For information, please write to SPECIAL SALES DEPARTMENT, Drelwood Communication Inc., P. O. Box 149, Indianola, WA 98342.

first printing 1992

Printed in the United States of America

This book is dedicated to all people who are taking the responsibility for maintaining health or recovering it through natural methods that include nutrition and exercise for the clear, inspired mind and soul of radiant health.

## ACKNOWLEDGMENTS

I wish to thank my instructors who through the written or spoken word on nutrition, preventive medicine, psychology, kinesiology, related sciences and philosophy have formed the basis for a better understanding of the Complete Person. And a heart-felt thank you to my audiences, my classes, to those who come to consult and to discuss. I learn the lion's share from you!

Elizabeth Baker, M.A.

# EATING, BELIEVING, ACHIEVING

*"And God said, Behold, I have given you every herb bearing seed, which is upon the face of all the earth, and every tree, in the which is the fruit of a tree yielding seed; to you it shall be for meat."*
Gen. 1-29  KJV

God's first commandment was how to eat. He wants us to treat our bodies with the utmost care. The body houses the spirit, His Holy Spirit, the entity that gives us a oneness with Him, our Father. We grieve the Holy Spirit when we do not follow God's commandment, a wrong-doing in His sight.

What is the meaning of that commandment? How do we follow it? By eating whole, all natural vegetables (herbs) for health and healing, the seeds (nuts, grains, legumes) for "meat" (the biblical meaning of "meat" is substance, not "flesh") and fruits with seeds. Technically, fruits are any seed-bearing pod that grows above ground, the "vine" in the Bible, as squash, tomato, bean, pea, eggplant, melon, etc. In fruits we get complete foods, rich in energy-giving calories.

By eating natural, unprocessed, mostly living foods, we get all the nutrients necessary to nourish our bodies for maximum function during a long, disease-free life, uplifted mind and spirit. Eating this way will naturally stabilize weight, taking off adipose (body fat) and keeping it off. In South Africa, where the natives eat unprocessed, natural foods, mostly raw, obesity, cancer, heart disease, arthritis, birth defects, emphysema, and so on are practically non-existent.

Weight loss diets of all kinds have come and gone, yet the problem of overweight goes on and on. We either eat to live or live to eat. Too often diets do not work for producing weight loss. What does work is a nutritional program designed to become a lifestyle for health, normal weight and high performance--physical, mental, emotional, spiritual. The seven phases of all natural foods in THE UN-DIET BOOK do work. The beautiful, delicious, satisfying, step-by-step, lifestyle laid out here brings us into the light of God's truth about eating of the abundance of His living foods. We have the choice of eating the all-natural way he intended, or the commercial, processed, depleted way man has created.

When we walk away from His plan for our life, we are diverted from self-discipline into indulgences and temptations that lead us astray. It is a downhill road taking little effort. At great cost in money, health and self esteem, it leads to wrong foods, overeating and weight gain. *"But the wages of sin is death,"* Romans 6:23.

When food consumption is not much in excess, the average person who tends to gain weight will add a pound a year. To project that rate of gain, a twenty-year old woman, 5'5" or 5'6" tall and weighing a beautiful 125 pounds, will weigh 145 pounds at age forty. At sixty years of age she will weigh 165 pounds which puts her in the class of the obese, all from eating more calories than are expended (burned by activity-exercise). *"And every man that striveth for the mastery is temperate in all things." 1 Corinthians 9:25 KJV*

There are several ways of eating an excess amount. The most common is simply eating too much at mealtime, a habit we may gradually and unconsciously cultivate. Laying down the fork or spoon between bites may well be the answer. Or serving the plates in the kitchen then not going for seconds. Or drinking a tall glass of water before each meal. One of the most effective ways to lessen the compulsion to overeat is to take low calorie, nutritional yeast in water or chilled herbal tea before a meal. It also cuts the appetite for more food by meeting deficiencies that cause cravings for calories. (Nutritional yeast does not contribute to candida albicans).

Another common weight-gain eating habit is snacking. A truly healthy person does not feel the need or desire to snack between meals. A snacker is often one who suffers from allergies and hypoglycemia. When he/she eliminates the cause of those allergies and corrects the deficiencies (usually minerals, vitamins and enzymes, abundant in raw foods) the need or desire for snacking is gone.

Then there is the closet eater. Although that may indicate a psychological or emotional problem, it can also indicate deficiencies that prompt cravings. For the person who has pricks of conscience, indulging in those cravings has to be as secret as possible. *"Set your affections on things above, not on things on the earth." Colossians 5:17 KJV*

Of course we all are aware of binging, an act that can contribute a great deal to overweight if indulged in frequently. Binging, too, can be an emotional/psychological problem. However, as with any eating disorder, binging oftentimes has as a basic cause, nutritional deficiencies. Usually, binge foods are sweets and fatty starches with perhaps chocolate at the head of the list. Chocolate binging may indicate a deficiency of the amino acid l-lysine. Binging on sugar sweets may indicate a deficiency of chromium, the glucose tolerance factor.

Many would have us believe it is all right to binge on sweets or other junk foods now and then. They go on to advise not to feel guilty. But shouldn't we feel guilty when we've done wrong? Not feeling guilty is part of the problem of not taking the responsibility for our life, for our own health. Such advice is unkind. It is permissive, indulgent. It is unwise. It is wrong.

Overeating (binging or eating too much at a meal, eating secretly, snacking at bedtime or nibbling while watching TV), creates a cruel overload for the body. It's like piling two or three times the normal pack load on a horse to go up the mountain. That toxic overload "winds" the body, breaks it down and eventually makes it sick. Many doctors believe overeating is the single, most harmful-to-the-health act in a normal person's normal day.

But take heart. There is a way out. Anyone can follow that way, a lifestyle that works, the lifestyle laid out and explained in THE UN-DIET BOOK. *"--Listen to me, and eat what is good, and your soul will delight in the richest of fare."* Isaiah 55:11 NIV

It is not difficult to plan daily to serve three highly nutritious, delicious and satisfying meals totaling 1200 to 1500 calories, sufficient for the average, active adult. The secret lies in raw foods which take a fraction of the body energy cooked and processed foods require for digestion.

It has been found raw fruits take only eight percent of the body's total energy to be digested. Raw vegetables require around twelve percent of total body energy, while unsprouted nuts and seeds (sunflower, sesame, pumpkin, etc.) utilize fifteen to twenty percent of total body energy.

By contrast, cooked and processed foods take from thirty to sixty-five percent of total body energy. This leaves much less energy for physical activity to burn up extra calories. The result is more adipose (weight). The undiet program--comfortable to follow, energy-giving, satisfying--allows for individual differences. *"Beloved, I wish above all things, that thou mayest prosper and be in health, even as thy soul prospereth."* III John 2 KJV

Changing a lifestyle takes faith in and commitment to our Creator. Without these we fail. Failure leads to discouragement, depression and eating for consolation and for emotional relief. Avoiding failure by commitment and trust, we begin to eat for health and enjoyment, for normal weight balance and stabilization. From that comes pleasure in eating and freedom from guilt. *"Bless the Lord---who satisfieth thy mouth with good things: so that thy youth is renewed like Eagle's."* Psalms 105 KJV

Wholehearted trust in Him for doing His will leads to the door of achievement. By this entrance into and work within His will, we enjoy good health, a normal-size body, peace of mind and a oneness with His Holy Spirit.

*"Then you will call upon me and come and pray to me and I will listen to you. And you will seek me and find me, when you search for me with all your heart."*
                                        *Jeremiah 29:12-13 NASB*

# Table of Contents

Introduction ........................................ 11

PART I The Transitional Diet Program ................... 13

Phase I. .......................................... 15

Phase II. ......................................... 27

Phase III. ........................................ 41

Phase IV. ......................................... 53

Phase V. .......................................... 65

Phase VI. ......................................... 75

Phase VII. ........................................ 87

PART II Transitional Guidelines for Your Health .......... 101

Chapter 1. A Clean Digestive System is Vital ............. 103

Chapter 2. Discover Your Allergies With Kinesiology Testing . 107

Chapter 3. How Processed Foods Bankrupt Your Health ..... 113

Chapter 4. Dynamic Natural Food Alternatives ........... 119

Chapter 5. What About Natural Food Supplements? ....... 123

Chapter 6. Kitchen Equipment That Works Magic ........ 127

Chapter 7. Make Your Kitchen Your Garden! ............. 131

Chapter 8. Multi-Miracles of Dehydrated Foods ........... 139

Chapter 9. Stable Emotions and a Positive Attitude ........ 143

PART III Transitional Recipes for a New You .. ............ 145

Appendix .......................................... 169

Glossary .......................................... 197

Bibliography ....................................... 201

Index ............................................. 203

# List of
# Charts and Tables

Sprouting Chart ...................................... 136

Table of Food Composition ............................. 180

Most Dangerous Food Additives ....................... 190

Convenient Equivalent Chart .......................... 193

# INTRODUCTION

Doctors continue to advocate a "balanced diet" as the foundation for good health. But what does a balanced diet really mean? Especially when the vast majority of food choices are nutritionally ravaged. Harmful additives, chemical alterations and artificial ingredients infest most of the goods on your supermarket shelf.

Yet in a world polluted by such foods, we can each survive in radiant health, clear mind and loving spirit! Countless people are taking their health management into their own hands and finding a way out of this nutritional desert. And rightfully so. Too long have we turned this privilege over to someone else. It is the responsibility of every one of us as thinking adults to study our own body and provide it with maximum health and freedom from disease!

Pursuing survival in today's world offers new opportunities for creative action. It involves avoiding bankrupt foods. And it means reeducating ourselves to become the complete, balanced person of body, mind and spirit God intended. Then we will have the strength not only to survive in our impure world, but to survive radiantly!

And what a wonderful help that God has told us what to eat for joy, health and robust longevity "...*every herb bearing seed, which is upon the face of all the earth, and every tree, in which is the fruit of a tree yielding seed;*" (Gen. 1:29) also "...*the tree of life, which bare twelve manner of fruits, and yielded her fruit every month; and the leaves of the tree were for the healing of the nations,*" (Rev. 2:22).

The Complete Person we all aspire to is symbolized by the triangle. The vital base is nutrition. One side represents our thinking; the other our physical well-being. To have a sturdy triangle we must eat properly--nurture spiritual, positive thoughts--and develop and preserve our bodies.

This is the thrust of THE UN-DIET BOOK. It offers an exciting path to an all-natural way to eat, think and exercise. Part I deals with the transitional diet program in seven easy Phases. Each Phase has a week's menus of simple-to-prepare, mostly inexpensive foods that balance the diet daily. They have been carefully researched to give you the greatest nutritional benefits. There are no "don'ts"; only constructive "dos". Not until the end of each Phase are you told what harmful food you deleted from your diet.

You can breeze through each Phase in a week, stay two weeks, or continue for several months. You move on only when you are ready. There's no pressure to do this or that, no hurry, nothing to make you feel guilty. And you don't need a gourmet-equipped, all-electric kitchen. In fact, we explain how you can grow many of the foods you eat right in your kitchen! They put money in your pocket and vigor in your body.

There are basic recipes, facts galore and helpful hints and explanations of what, why and where to buy each week for your new health-giving menus. Also included are inspiring messages and a program of exercise leading to optimal health.

The chapters in Part II spell out how to maintain-- or regain-- health. They are simple. They are direct. They are fun. Since they come from our Creator, we can trust and follow them and know that we will triumph. Welcome to a new world of gastronomical enjoyment and a healthier, happier, more Complete New You!

Elizabeth Baker

# The
## Transitional
### Diet Program

# Phase I

*"And out of the ground made the Lord God to grow every tree that is pleasant to the sight, and good for food..."*

*Genesis 2:9*

You are started! You're on your way to an exciting new adventure. Here's your first step: use only stainless steel, cast iron, Corningware, fireproof glassware or enamel for cooking. Do not use copper or aluminum which dissolve into the food, or coated utensils which are petrochemically treated and gas off in the foods. When you buy any processed or prepared foods, be sure to read the labels for harmful additives to avoid (see Appendix) and buy those with the fewest preservatives, artificial color, sugar, flavor and other chemicals.

New, unconventional dishes appearing in the following menus are numbered thus: (1), (2), (3), etc. Recipes for them appear under the corresponding number at the end of each Phase.

Recipes are for four persons unless otherwise stated. Lunches are for home, office, work, school, for a quick, simple picnic or to take to a sick friend or relative in a rest home or hospital. They are for one person.

For your convenience we include here the abbreviations of measurements used in the recipes that follow.

| | | |
|---|---|---|
| C. = cup | pt. = pint | lb. = pound |
| T. = tablespoon | qt. = quart | oz. = ounce |
| t. = teaspoon | gal. = gallon | |

## Special Foods Shopping List

Here is a list of special foods you may not customarily have in your kitchen. They can be found in grocery stores, supermarkets, co-ops, natural grain stores, health food stores and farmer-type markets.

| | | |
|---|---|---|
| Jack cheese | Vegetable spaghetti | Rumford's Baking |
| Wheat bran | Molasses | Powder |
| Honey (raw) | Rye bread | Skim (non-fat) milk |
| Pocket bread | Whole wheat bread | Cinnamon bark |
| Carob | Wheat bran | |

| | | |
|---|---|---|
| Barley malt syrup | Vegetable salt | Honey-granola-bars |
| Apple cider vinegar | Sodium Ascorbate | or dried figs |
| Spice tea | (S.A.) (see | Brown rice |
| | Appendix) | |

# Daily Menus

## Monday

**Breakfast:** Bacon and eggs
Toast and date jam (1)

Grapefruit
Black coffee, tea or skim milk

**Lunch:** Whole wheat sandwich with mayonnaise and jack cheese

Celery sticks
Apple
Black coffee or skim milk

**Dinner:** Pot roast with vegetables
Bran muffins (2)
Honey butter (3)

Fresh radishes
Bowl of raisins and peanuts
Black coffee, tea, milk

*Do ahead: Soak prunes for Tuesday*

## Tuesday

**Breakfast:** Scrambled eggs
Toast

Prunes
Black coffee or milk

**Lunch:** Pocket Bread with peanut butter (4)
Black coffee or Chocarob (5)

Carrot sticks
Grapes

**Dinner:** Roast pork, well done
Sweet potatoes
Gravy
Spice tea or milk

Lettuce salad with grated zucchini
Wheat bread, margarine or butter
Date whip (6)

## Wednesday

**Breakfast:** Oatmeal with raisins and barley malt syrup
Toast melba

Orange juice
Black coffee or milk

**Lunch:** Crackers and cheese (naturally aged or Jack cheese)
Fruit juice

Cabbage wedge
Honey-granola bar (available at health-food store) or dried figs

**Dinner:** Vegetable spaghetti and meat balls

Spinach salad with your favorite dressing

Buttered broccoli  
Black coffee, tea or milk

Bread sticks  
Fresh grapes

## Thursday

**Breakfast:** Whole wheat pancakes, molasses, honey or barley malt syrup  
Sausages (fresh ground)

Apple juice, unsweetened  
Black coffee, tea or milk

**Lunch:** Tuna-on-rye sandwich with lettuce  
Black coffee, buttermilk or yogurt

Zucchini sticks  
Dates

**Dinner:** Rice casserole with chopped beef (8)  
Buttered peas  
Fresh fruit in season

Sliced tomato and cucumber salad (7)  
Whole wheat bread  
Raisin jam (9)  
Black coffee, tea or milk

*Do ahead: Soak prunes for Friday.*

## Friday

**Breakfast:** English muffins  
Soft boiled eggs, sprinkled with bran

Pineapple juice, natural  
Black coffee, tea or milk

**Lunch:** Mashed brown or pinto beans and bean sprouts sandwich on multi-grain bread

Cucumber slices  
Pear  
Black coffee, tea or buttermilk

**Dinner:** Meat loaf  
Baked potato  
Buttered beets  
Black coffee, tea or milk

Green salad  
Hot rolls  
Prune whip (10)

## Saturday

**Breakfast:** Bran waffles or pancakes  
Berry-date syrup (11)

Ham  
Cantaloupe or fruit in season  
Black coffee, tea or milk

*Do ahead: Soak 1 C. chopped figs for Saturday lunch.*

**Lunch:** Brown or navy bean soup  
Cornbread  
Black coffee, tea or milk

Fig jam (12)  
Fresh fruit

**Dinner:** Oven fried chicken
Mashed potatoes
Gravy
Blueberry or raisin muffins
(13)
Black coffee, tea or milk

Cauliflower with grated
parmesan cheese
Waldorf salad (14)
Apple crisp (15)

## Sunday

**Breakfast:** Unsweetened dry cereal with
raisins, dates or bananas
Toast with nut butter (16)

Pineapple or prune juice
Black coffee, tea or milk

**Dinner:** Mid day
Roast turkey legs
Chinese stir-fried vegetables
Sliced tomatoes

Brown rice
Honey-rice cookies (17)
Tea, milk

**Supper:** Hot Chocarob (drink) made
with milk and carob
powder)
Popcorn

Fresh fruit in season
Nuts, unroasted

Congratulations! You have gotten through a week without sugar, a major accomplishment! Of course sugar masquerades in several different forms—corn syrup, dextrose, etc.

If you wish to continue with just taking *sugar* out of your diet, you may want to turn to the "Sweets and Desserts" in PART III, TRANSITIONAL RECIPES to satisfy everyone's sweet tooth. Most of us in the Western hemisphere are sugar addicts, making it difficult to cut out white table sugar. But you will find, as time goes on and you get more complete nourishment, you will gradually crave fewer and fewer sweets.

Have dates, apple leather, raisins, figs, and/or Frozen Bananas (see recipe in Part III) and pure, fresh, cold water in easy reach for quick serving so no one will be tempted to run to a refreshment stand for a sweet soft drink or candy bar.

On rare occasions or for very special treats, serve a bowl of natural carob chips with nuts, peanuts or Buckwheat Crunchies. Chocolate addicts can "binge" occasionally on carob chips (made without sugar), found at health food stores and even supermarkets. Some contain date sugar.

When favorite foods such as conventional cakes, pies, cookies, bakery goods and candies are suddenly eliminated from the diet, many people become somewhat insecure. They honestly feel they'll go hungry. Take care of this understandable problem by providing plenty of substitutes, including sweet herbal teas, such as licorice, cinnamon bark or carob. At the end of a meal, these teas satisfy the craving for sweets. Or add a spoonful of barley malt syrup or molasses to milk or fruit juice. There are many ways of satisfying a sweet tooth without using sugar.

At all cost keep the family from refined white table sugar. Or, in other words, keep all sugar and sugar foods out of the house. Keep in mind this long-known truth: the less refined sugar in the diet, the better the brain functions.

Also, along the way there were opportunities for you to change little things. For instance, butter instead of margarine, and whole wheat products instead of devitalized white flour products. You might be surprised that there is hidden sugar in a lot of products, such as catsup, salad dressings, some crackers and breads, etc.

With your upswing in health will naturally come an upturn in your mental attitude, your inner spirit, your outlook on life. Take advantage of it and give thanks to God for guiding you. Ask for continual growth, positive philosophy and faith. You'll find you'll be less critical and more understanding of others, more patient and loving, less prone to anger or irritability.

## Exercise for Radiant Health

The hunting for, and preparation of, natural foods kept the ancients physically active and strong. Since we no longer have to bestir ourselves to all that effort and activity, we too often become sedentary and physically sluggish . . . conditions that contribute greatly to ill health and disease. To change all that, we must have muscle strength and good circulation. That means exercise daily or at least several times a week.

We are going to start you out on an easy, uncomplicated program of exercise that costs nothing, needs no regular, manufactured health equipment, special room or extra space. Do the exercises at your convenience. When you get up in the morning or you take a mid-morning or mid-afternoon or before-dinner break, or before you go to bed at night, do the following stretch exercises:

1. Out-of-doors or before an open window, stand straight with feet eight or 10 inches apart. Exhale, pushing all the air out of your lungs. Then as you start to inhale, begin stretching your hands straight out from the sides of your body to up over your head to a slow count of ten. Then exhale on a count of ten as you bring them down, straight out from your body, to your sides. Relax. Repeat two or three times. Do *not* overdo. Too much new exercise is painful and harmful.

2. Take a deep breath, then with hands and arms hanging limp, slowly bend down on a count of ten, as far as a comfortable stretch allows, touching your toes or the floor if possible.

Slowly rise back up, arms limp. Do three times.

3. Standing straight, take a deep breath, extend one arm up, one down and to a count of ten bring the one arm down as you bring the other up while you exhale. Raise and lower each extended, well-stretched arm two or three times. If this last stretch exercise begins to tire you unduly, do it only once or twice the first day.

Continue each exercise for a week or two, gradually increasing the number of times for each every day or two. Never overdo. Only you can tell when you've done enough. Just remember to increase a little bit every day or so until you get up to ten times for each one. Many find they can reach the ten times for each exercise in a week.

## Recipes for Phase I in the Order of Appearance

### 1. DATE JAM

1 C. pitted dates

½ C. warm water

Soak dates in warm water for an hour. Mix in a blender or mash and whip with a fork until creamy-smooth. You may need to add enough water to make a heavy cream. Chill and serve. (It will be quite thick.) Keep refrigerated.

### 2. BRAN MUFFINS

1½ C. flour, all-purpose

1 C. wheat bran

½ t. salt

2 t. baking powder

2 eggs

3 T. oil

1⅓ C. water

Mix dry ingredients. Make a cup-size hole in center of flour and add eggs, oil and water. Mix well. Bake at 350° in muffin pans or 9" x 9" pan for 35 (muffin pans) to 40 (square pan) minutes, or until lightly browned and the sides of muffins pull away from pan.

## 3. HONEY BUTTER

2 T. butter (room
   temperature)

1 C. raw honey

Mix the butter and honey together. Whip or blend to a thick cream and serve.


## 4. PEANUT BUTTER POCKET BREAD
### (Serves 1)

1 pocket bread

1 T. heaping, alfalfa sprouts

1 t. water

2 T. peanut butter

Chop the sprouts and mix with peanut butter and water. Fill the cut-opened pocket bread, spreading the mixture out. Serve.


## 5. HOT CHOCAROB

⅓ C. carob powder

1 C. milk (raw); or 1 C.
   reconstituted whey or 1
   scant C. water with 1 t.
   butter or 1 T. cream

1 or 2 drops vanilla

½ t. honey (optional)

Mix carob, vanilla and honey in milk, whey or water. Heat in double boiler or pan set in a larger pan of hot, not boiling, water. Stir well. Serves one person.


## 6. DATE WHIP

1 C. pitted dates

4 or 6 T. water or fruit juice

2 ripe bananas

Chop dates and soak in water fifteen minutes. Mash and whip with bananas, or blend all with a bit more liquid. Chill and serve with a dollop of cream, whipped or plain, or a sprinkle of unsweet coconut.

# 7. TOMATO-CUCUMBER SALAD

2 tomatoes (medium)

1 cucumber

4 T. sour cream

½ t. vegetable salt

Slice tomatoes and cucumber in shallow bowl. Spread sour cream over it and sprinkle with vegetable salt.

# 8. RICE CASSEROLE WITH CHOPPED BEEF

2 C. cooked, salted brown rice

1 T. butter

1 C. chopped mushrooms

1 C. fine-chopped celery

1 T. chopped onion (optional)

1½ C. cooked, diced beef

Dash pepper

Warm the rice. Add the butter, then all the ingredients, mixing with a lifting action to keep from packing the rice. Heat over hot water or in a low-heated oven. Do not boil or bake. You may be surprised at not having to cook the casserole. But be assured it is delicious hot with the crunchy, crisp vegetables.

# 9. RAISIN JAM

1 C. raisins

6 to 8 t. warm water

Fine-chop or grind raisins and mix with water, then mash with potato masher. Or blend, using double the amount of water. Chill and serve. Keep refrigerated.

# 10. PRUNE WHIP

1 C. pitted prunes

1 C. warm water

¼ C. orange or apple juice

Soak pitted prunes a few hours. Chop and mash, adding the fruit juice, and whip with fork. Or blend, adding ½ C. juice. Chill and serve topped with cream or chopped nuts or sesame seeds.

## 11.  BERRY-DATE SYRUP

¾ C. pitted, chopped dates

1 C. of any fresh or frozen berries

Mix chopped dates with mashed fruit and blend. Or mash thoroughly by hand. If syrup is too tart, add from 1 to 3 t. honey. The fruit syrup can be warmed over hot water to serve on hot waffles or pancakes.

## 12.  FIG JAM

1 C. cut-up, soaked figs

½ C. fig soak water or fruit juice

Soak figs a few hours in 1 C. water. Chop then blend with fig soak water and/or juice. Or mash to a thick cream. Chill and serve. Keep refrigerated.

## 13.  BLUEBERRY-BUCKWHEAT (OR RAISIN) MUFFINS

2 C. buckwheat flour

4 t. baking powder (use Rumford or similar brand without aluminum)

½ t. salt or 1½ t. S. A.

1¾ C. water

2 eggs

2 T. oil or melted butter

1 T. molasses

¾ C. blueberries, fresh or frozen, thawed and drained, or raisins or dehydrated blueberries plus 1 T. water

Mix together flour, baking powder, salt or S.A. In the depressed center of the flour mixture, pour in water, eggs, molasses, oil or butter and the blueberries or raisins. Stir. Spoon into lined muffin pans and bake at 375° or until lightly browned. Or bake in 9" x 9" pan at 375° for 35 minutes. Serve warm.

# 14. WALDORF SALAD

2 C. chopped, unpeeled apples

2 C. chopped celery

¾ C. chopped walnuts

½ C. grapes or raisins

¾ C. mayonnaise

1 T. honey

1 t. vinegar

1 sprig parsley

Lightly toss all together and serve or chill before serving. Garnish with parsley.

# 15. APPLE CRISP

6 apples, sliced

1 T., rounded, cornstarch

1 small can frozen apple juice

½ t. mace

1½ C. oatmeal

¼ t. cinnamon

¼ t. nutmeg

4 T. butter

Slice apples into a 9-inch square casserole or deep dish pie plate. Dissolve cornstarch in thawed apple juice. Pour over apples, sprinkle with mace. Mix crumbled oatmeal, cinnamon, nutmeg and bits of butter and spread over the apple mixture. Bake at 350° for 25 minutes. Cool, cut and serve, with or without whipped cream.

*Note: This can be made with success in a crock-pot.*

# 16. NUT BUTTER

1 C. nuts (any kind)

2 to 3 T. oil or water

Finely chop nuts and put through a seed-nut mill. Or spread on a cookie sheet or flat baking pan and with a wooden rolling pin, roll until nuts are in fine particles. Or grind in food grinder. Place meal in bowl, add water or oil to make a room-temperature butter consistency. Chill for a firmer nut butter. Keep refrigerated.

# 17. RICE COOKIES

1½ C. well-cooked warm, brown, salted rice

3 t. baking powder

2 eggs

2 T. water

2 T. melted butter or vegetable oil

1 C. unsweet coconut

1 t. vanilla

Mash the rice with potato masher, sprinkle baking powder over it, add the other ingredients and mix well with spoon or by hand to a stiff dough. Drop in 2-inch circles on oiled cookie sheet or pat in an 8" x 11" oiled, glass baking dish. Bake 15 to 20 minutes at 350° or until golden brown. Cut in 2½ inch squares when cooled to slightly warm. Store in tightly lidded containers. Cookies are chewy.

# Phase II

*"Beloved, I wish above all things that thou mayest prosper and be in health, even as thy soul prospereth."*
                                        III John 2

When you feel comfortable with the Phase I diet and you find your appetite is doing quite well with no table sugar in foods, you are ready for Phase II. You may have been on the first phase for one week or two months. The time to move on to the next phase is when you feel psychologically, emotionally and physically ready to continue with the change.

Phase II's differences are slight and subtle, but far-reaching in your progress toward health. Their importance cannot be over-stressed. Here are the menus prepared for that progress. Carry on. Trust and hold faith.

## Special Foods Shopping List

Sunflower seeds (hulled)
Dried apples
Tortillas (frozen or fresh)
Mint tea
Buttermilk
Buckwheat flour
Puffed rice crackers
Dates, date sugar and/or date bits
Whey powder

Camomile tea
Comfrey tea
Lemon grass tea
Shave grass tea
Barley flour
Vegetable or whole wheat macaroni
Jack cheese
Avocado
Yams
Lentils

Cornmeal
Granola (with honey)
Blueberries or raisins
Hierba Mate
Oil, cold pressed (see Glossary)
Millet
Dill weed
Salad seasoning (mix)

## Daily Menus

### Monday

**Breakfast:**  Scrambled eggs
Dried apple jam (1)
Black coffee, tea or skim milk

Buttered toast
Fresh fruit in season, or juice

*Do ahead: Soak ½ C. sunflower seeds for Tuesday breakfast. In the evening, drain, wash and allow to drain. Refrigerate.*

**Lunch:** Salad tacos (2)  
Raw nuts (any kind)  

Banana  
Mint tea or buttermilk

**Dinner:** Poached fish (any kind)  
Lemon butter sauce (3)  
Buckwheat stove-top  
muffins  
Butter  
Orange date marmalade  

Eden or frozen corn (4)  
Spinach salad and vinegar  
dressing (5)  
Orange slices  
Lemon grass tea (7)

*Do ahead: Soak for sprouting: 2 tablespoons of alfalfa or mung beans for Friday.*

## Tuesday

**Breakfast:** Oatmeal with sunflower  
seeds (8)  
Toast with butter  

Fresh fruit in season  
Black coffee, tea or skim  
milk

**Lunch:** Puffed rice crackers and  
peanut butter served with  
chopped dates (9)  
Carrot sticks  

Apple  
Camomile tea, cold or hot,  
with or without honey

**Dinner:** Creamed dried beef (10)  
Buttered broccoli  
Zucchini-romaine-tomato  
salad  

Oil and vinegar salad  
dressing  
Rolls and honey  
Grapes  
Black coffee, tea or skim  
milk

## Wednesday

**Breakfast:** French toast with whole  
wheat bread  
Fig jam  
Butter  

Grapefruit or juice  
Black coffee, hot whey, or tea

*Do ahead: Sprout 1 C. lentils for Saturday. (See Chapter 7 for sprouting table.)*

**Lunch:** Glass-packed fish or poached  
fish sandwich with leaf  
lettuce  
Olives, celery sticks  

Oatmeal-coconut-raisin  
cookies (11)  
Comfrey-spice tea (12)

**Dinner:** Chili beans and ground beef Cucumber-tomato-avocado
Corn stove-top muffins (13)   salad
Hierba mate tea   Date-nut plate

*Do ahead: In a large bowl, mix the barley flour and yeast for tomorrow's breakfast pancakes (recipe 14). Cover with a cloth. Do not refrigerate.*

## Thursday

**Breakfast:** Barley flour pancakes (14) Small, lean, broiled
Butter malt syrup (15)   hamburger
Black coffee, comfrey-mint Fresh fruit in season
  tea or skim milk

**Lunch:** Deviled egg-on-rye Banana
  sandwich Camomile-clove tea or skim
Celery sticks, dill pickle   milk

**Dinner:** Vegetable or whole wheat Reconstituted dried
  macaroni made with Jack   apricots, pears, peaches or
  cheese (16)   apples or any combination
Buttered peas and carrots   of them
Coconut cookies Black coffee, spearmint tea,
  or skim milk

## Friday

**Breakfast:** Soft-boiled eggs (2 minutes) Whole wheat cinnamon
  sprinkled with toast   toast with butter
  crumbs Coffee, lemon grass tea or
Prunes, reconstituted, or   skim milk
  fresh fruit in season

**Lunch:** Almond paste tacos (17) Cinnamon-carob tea (19)
Yam sticks (18)

**Dinner:** Millet-Walnut Casserole Whole wheat bread
  (20) Carrot cake (22)
Buttered beets with tops (21) Black coffee, spiced tea or
Coleslaw   skim milk

## Saturday

**Breakfast:** Oatmeal pancakes with Apple Juice
  honey Shave grass tea or hot whey
Soft scrambled eggs   drink

**Lunch:** Lentil soup (23) Green salad with guacamole
Corn bread   dressing (24)
Butter, molasses Black coffee, comfrey-mint
  tea or buttermilk

| **Dinner:** | Broiled lamb or ground steak | Sliced tomatoes |
| | Baked potato with butter or | Rye bread |
| | sour cream | Frozen bananas |
| | Green beans | Coffee, hierba mate tea, or |
| | | skim milk |

## Sunday

| **Breakfast:** | Granola cereal with cream or | Cantaloupe |
| | fruit juice | Black coffee, shave grass tea, |
| | Cracked wheat blueberry | skim milk |
| | muffins | |

| **Dinner:** | Chicken and dumplings | Fresh fruit in season with |
| | Buttered cauliflower | raisin cookies |
| | Waldorf salad | Black coffee, camomile tea or |
| | | skim milk |

| | Popcorn | Carob-whey drink |
| **Supper:** | Bananas | |

BRAVO! You have just eliminated hard fats and processed oils! They are probably the second greatest contribution to ill health, sugar being the first. Now you can enjoy the improved feeling of well-being, and the taste of the natural, raw, nourishing, fresh oils and seeds, nuts, avocado and sweet, raw cow butter.

Besides these sweet fats, you have added millet, dried apple jam, lemon-butter sauce for your fish, raw, buttered roasting ears or fresh or frozen corn, stove-top corn and buckwheat muffins, barley malt syrup, rice cakes, yam sticks, frozen bananas, shave grass tea, and more.

You can plan to carry on in Phase II for days, weeks or months before the next change—or proceed immediately to Phase III. It's an easy one.

Count your blessings. Smile a lot. Anticipate the new adventure of learning to experience an all-natural diet and improved health.

# Exercises for Phase II

The exercises are mild but so effective against tension in the head, shoulders and neck. They also promote clearer thinking... all-important in today's busy, competitive world.

1. The Head Roll—Sitting up straight in a comfortable, back-supporting, hard chair, take a deep breath, exhale, then drop the head down (forward) as if fallen asleep. Now roll the head slowly to the left shoulder, on to the back (keeping mouth closed), then to the right shoulder and to the chest. The neck should be limp, the shoulders relaxed. Roll the head around

in this circle two or three times, breathing deeply to a count of ten as you do so. Then sit a moment enjoying the feeling of relaxation.

2. Again, inhale to a count of ten as you slowly drop the head forward, as though in dead sleep. Then exhaling, slowly raise the head until it is leaning back over the shoulders. All to a count of ten. Do two or three times, then relax in normal sit-up position.

3. Hunch the shoulders and turn the head back and forth against the hunched shoulders. This is a wonderful, natural massage.

Add these three simple, effective exercises to those of Phase I and do each day. Astronauts, truck drivers, business executives, housewives—all find these three little exercises among the top most effective for relaxation and a clear head.

## Recipes for Phase II

## 1. DRIED APPLE JAM

2 C. dried apples

1 small can frozen apple juice

water

Soak the apples in the thawed juice and enough more water to barely cover the apples when pressed down. Blend or mash and whip to a cream. Serve. Keep refrigerated.

## 2. SALAD TACOS
## (Serves 4 people)

8 untoasted corn tortillas

Butter

1 avocado (large)

1 T. vinegar or lemon juice

1½ t. S.A. or ½ t. salt

Dash or two salad seasoning

Alfalfa or bean sprouts

Brush tortillas with soft butter. Peel and mash avocado then mix in vinegar or lemon juice and seasonings. Spread on tortillas, sprinkle generously with sprouts, roll into inch-and-a-half tubes and secure with toothpicks.

## 3. LEMON BUTTER SAUCE
### (for poached fish)

1 C. fish broth

1 T. (rounded) cornstarch

2 T. water

2 T. butter

1½ T. lemon juice

   Dash paprika

   Dash pepper

1½ t. S.A. or salt

Moisten cornstarch with water and add to boiling fish broth, stirring until thickened. (About a minute.) Set aside to cool slightly—about 2 minutes. Add butter, lemon juice and seasonings, stirring well. Serve over fish.

## 4. EDEN CORN # 1

4 fresh ears of corn

   Large pot of water

*Note: We heat and serve the corn in Fireproop Pyrex or Corningware.*

Heat water to about 140°. (You can't quite put your hand on the pan.) Do not boil. Submerge corn and let sit 5 minutes. Place on low heat until as hot as your fingers can endure (115° to 120°). Serve with butter in pre-heated, covered vegetable dish, or directly onto the plates from the hot kettle of water.

## EDEN CORN # 2

1 12 oz. package frozen corn or 1½ C. fresh, cut-off corn. (Be sure to scrape cob to include the kernel.)

½ t. salt (optional)

½ C. water

1 T. butter

Thaw corn, or cut corn off the cob. Boil the cobs for 5 minutes in water. When slightly cooled, pour this water and corn in double boiler, or pan set in hot water, add salt and butter and serve in pre-heated vegetable dish.

*Note: Corn served heated but uncooked is so super delicious you'll never cook it again. Your family and guests will love it! (Don't tell them it's uncooked until you've served it several times. Then and only then, reveal your secret.) Corn thus prepared and/or blended with 120° to 140° water and butter becomes our favorite cream soup.*

## 5. SPINACH SALAD, VINEGAR DRESSING

¼ C. cold pressed salad oil

¼ C. vinegar or lemon juice

Salad seasoning, your own favorite (or see Part III recipes)

Make your favorite green salad using spinach instead of lettuce. Mix all the ingredients listed here in a bottle, shake and toss with the salad.

## 6. BUCKWHEAT STOVE-TOP MUFFINS

2 C. buckwheat flour

3 t. baking powder

1½ t. S. A. or ½ t. salt

2 eggs

1¾ C. water

2 T. oil

Mix dry ingredients then add the others and stir well. The batter will be thicker than pancake batter to make a firmer, thicker, muffin-like cake. Bake on slightly oiled iron griddle or skillet in 3-inch circles. These delicious, firm, heavy, chewy muffins can be eaten with the hand as an oven baked muffin. We put our stainless steel, electric skillet on a TV table set by the table and bake and serve as family or friends eat them, fresh and hot.

## 7. LEMON GRASS TEA
## (Children love it!)

3 t. lemon grass, rounded or 3 bags

4 C. boiling water

½ T. ascorbic acid powder (vitamin C) or 1 T. lemon juice

4 t. honey

Pour water over tea in a pot or pan, cover and let steep 5 to 10 minutes. Strain or remove bags. Stir in the vitamin C or lemon juice and honey and serve. Delicious as ice cold tea.

# 8. OATMEAL-SUNFLOWER CEREAL

2 C. oatmeal

1¾ C. hot water

1 t. salt

¾ C. raisins

¾ C. budded sunflower
seeds

4 t. honey or molasses
(optional)

Put oatmeal, salt and water in pan, bring to a full boil, stir slightly, top with tight lid, turn off heat and let sit 3 or 4 minutes. Remove from burner and allow to cool slightly. Add raisins and honey or molasses. Serve with milk, cream, butter or fruit juice.

# 9. RICE CAKE-PEANUT BUTTER MUNCHIES

4 large, puffed rice cakes

4 T. peanut butter

4 T. date sugar or ½ C.
chopped dates

Mix peanut butter and dates or date sugar and spread on the rice cakes for a special treat.

# 10. CREAMED DRIED BEEF

1½ T. butter

3 T. whole wheat flour

¼ t. salt

Dash of cayenne

1 C. milk, reconstituted
whey or water plus 3 T.

1 C. dried beef

Melt butter, add flour, salt and cayenne and stir. Add half the milk, stirring until it thickens and boils, then the other half, stirring until it boils. Cut or tear dried beef in small pieces and add to the white sauce. Bring to a boil and serve.

*Note: For a most unusual, super white sauce, blend ¾ C. unsweetened coconut, fresh or dried, with 1 C. and 2 T. of warm water, strain and use to make the sauce. If fresh coconut is left over, serve it at another meal instead of nuts or budded sunflower seeds, or blend with twice as much water, strain to make coconut milk. Serve over oatmeal. A real taste thrill!*

# 11. OATMEAL COCONUT COOKIES

2 C. oatmeal

1½ t. S.A. or ½ t. salt

2 t. baking powder

1 C. grated, unsweetened coconut

1 C. raisins

1 egg

¾ C. water

3 T. oil

3 T. honey

Mix together dry ingredients, raisins and coconut. In the indented center of the dry mixture, drop the egg, water, oil and honey. Stir to a stiff batter. Drop by spoonfuls on an oiled cookie sheet and bake at 350° for 25 minutes, or until a very light brown.

# 12. COMFREY SPICE TEA

4 t. comfrey, heaping

Dash each of clove, cinnamon and nutmeg

¼ t. of broken bits of dried orange peel or grated rind

4 C. boiling water

Put all ingredients in a pan. Add boiling water, cover and steep for 5 minutes. Strain into teapot or thermos. It is delicious served as iced tea.

# 13. CORN STOVE-TOP MUFFINS

2 C. yellow cornmeal

3 t. baking powder

1½ t. S.A. or ½ t. salt

2 T. oil or melted butter

2 eggs

1½ C. water

Mix corn meal, baking powder and salt then add oil or butter, eggs and water, stirring to a rather stiff batter. Bake on griddle or skillet, slightly oiled, in 3-inch circles, until golden brown on each side. Serve at once.

# 14. BARLEY PANCAKES

1 T., rounded, dry bread yeast

½ C. lukewarm water

2 C. barley flour

1½ t. S.A. or ½ t. salt

1 egg

3 T. oil

1¼ C. water at room temperature

Dissolve yeast in lukewarm water and set aside in warm place. Mix dry ingredients and water and set aside for over night. Before breakfast, stir down the batter, add egg and oil and stir well. Set aside while you prepare the rest of breakfast. The batter will rise some. You can carefully spoon out batter and onto the oiled skillet or grill, retaining some of the lightness. Or stir the batter down, and proceed as with ordinary pancakes. Serve as they are baked.

# 15. BUTTER MALT SYRUP

1 C. barley malt syrup

2 T. hot water

2 T. butter

Warm the barley malt syrup in a pan set in hot water. Add water and butter, stir well and serve over barley pancakes.

# 16. MACARONI WITH CHEESE

1½ C. vegetable macaroni

3 C. boiling water

1 t. salt

1 C. grated jack cheese or uncolored (white) cheddar

1 C. white sauce made with whole wheat flour

Dash of cayenne

Chopped parsley

Cook macaroni and salt in the water until tender. Drain. Spread evenly in a baking dish, pour the white sauce over it, then sprinkle the cheese on top. Bake at 325° until cheese is melted, and serve with parsley dotted over it.

# 17. ALMOND PASTE TACOS

1 C. almonds

½ t. S.A. (if you want it to keep several days)

3 or 4 T. water

Grind the almonds finely, in grinder or seed mill. Add S.A. and water to make a thick paste. Spread on tortillas. Salt to taste. Sprinkle with sprouts—watercress, radish, clover, alfalfa or bean. Roll in tubes, stick with toothpicks and wrap for brown bag lunch, picnic or serve at once.

# 18. YAM STICKS
## (So sweet and crisp!)

1 fresh yam

Scrub yam with stiff brush. Do not peel. Cut lengthwise in 1-inch wide sticks. Serve as a relish or with a nut butter dip.

# 19. CINNAMON CAROB TEA (1 C.)

1 T. (heaping) carob

1 T. (heaping) powdered whey

¼ t. cinnamon

¾ C. very hot water

1 drop vanilla

½ t. butter (optional)

Mix dry ingredients together, add hot water, vanilla and butter. Stir well and serve.

# 20. MILLET-WALNUT CASSEROLE

1 C. millet

2 C. boiling water

½ t. salt

2 T. butter

¾ C. walnuts, broken bits

Pour water over millet and salt, bring to a boil, cover, turn burner on simmer for 30 minutes. Turn off heat and leave pan on burner for several minutes. Set aside to cool slightly, then add butter and walnuts. Stir carefully to keep millet fluffy. Serve in pre-heated dish.

## 21. BUTTERED BEETS WITH TOPS

1 bunch fresh beets and tops

1 C. boiling water

1 T. butter

½ t. salt

Steam beets until tender, cool, remove skins and dice. Separately steam beet tops 2 or 3 minutes. Chop and combine with beets, butter and salt. Reheat if desired, and serve.

## 22. CARROT CAKE

2 C. whole wheat flour

4 t. baking powder

½ t. salt or 1½ t. S.A.

½ t. mace

¼ t. allspice

2 C. grated carrots

2 eggs

4 T. honey

3 T. oil

¾ C. chopped dates

½ C. chopped nuts

½ t. vanilla

1 C. (scant) water

Mix dry ingredients together, Add the rest in order given. Blend all well. Pour into oiled 8½" x 11" baking dish and bake at 350° for 40 minutes. The cake will slightly stick to a dry toothpick when inserted. Allow to cool in the dish, cutting out and serving while still warm.

## 23. SPROUTED LENTIL SOUP (No. 1)

2 C. lentil sprouts

1 t. salt or 1½ t. S.A. and ½ t. salt

2 C. water

2 T. butter

1 T. chopped celery

1 T. chopped onion (optional)

Place 1½ cups lentil sprouts in soup pan and cook in the water for ten minutes. Set aside to cool to 140°. (You can almost hold your hand on bottom of pan.) Add salt, butter, chopped celery and onion. If cooled too much, heat to 120° on low burner. Add the ½ cup raw sprouts and serve in heated soup cups.

*Note: When lentils and beans are sprouted they lose their gas-causing factor. 1 C. of lentils or beans yields about 2 C. sprouts, packed-in-the-cup measure.*

# 24. GUACAMOLE

1 avocado

1 T. vinegar or lemon juice

2 T. water

¼ t. celery salt

¼ t. dill weed

Peel and mash avocado to a cream. Add vinegar or lemon juice, water and seasonings. Mix and serve over a green salad or as a dip for crackers or vegetable sticks.

*Note: Guacamoles are like people. No two are alike. Seasonings make the difference.*

# Phase III

*" . . . to make a distinction between the unclean and the clean, and between the edible creature and the creature which is not to be eaten."*

*Leviticus 11:47*

At this point you will have little difficulty in proceeding in the transitional period of your next food changes. If you regress now and then, don't spend time and emotional energy in giving yourself a bad time. Just ask God to give you His help and strength to succeed. He will. Then give thanks. Smile at yourself, take a deep breath and study your next menu. It's simply delicious!

Don't look beyond making your grocery lists for the next week and to putting sunflower seeds and lentils to soak. You'll find yourself saving money and spending less time in the kitchen cooking and in scrubbing up after meals.

Carry on and praise God!

## Special Foods List

Jícama (see Glossary)
Cranberries (if autumn)
Pocket bread
Wasa bread or Zwieback
Hibiscus (Jamaica) tea (see Glossary)

Buckwheat noodles
Rabbit
Honey graham crackers
White cheddar cheese
Sweet potatoes
Barley flour

Sesame seeds, natural
Sassafras tea
Tofu (see Glossary)
Rice bran
Pumpkin seeds
Sunflower seeds, raw, hulled
Whey powder

## Daily Menus

### Monday

**Breakfast:** Cooked whole grain cereal with cream or butter, nuts and honey if desired

Bananas
Black coffee, tea or skim milk

*Do ahead: Soak 1 cup of lentils for Wednesday lunch.*

41

**Lunch:** Drained cottage cheese on buttered rye bread layered with bean or alfalfa sprouts and eaten as an open face sandwich or on a platter eaten with a fork
Mint tea or fruit juice

Jícama or turnip slice and/or cherry tomatoes
Whole wheat carob chip cookies (Make your favorite chocolate chip cookie recipe, substituting whole wheat flour for white flour, carob chips for chocolate chips. For the sugar, substitute honey or molasses using half as much since both are twice as sweet as sugar.)

**Dinner:** Salmon, tuna, or white fish mixed in scalloped potatoes
Green beans, buttered
Green salad with avocado dressing

Whole wheat bread
Pumpkin pie made with honey as sugar
Black coffee, comfrey tea or skim milk

*Do ahead: Soak ⅔ cup of almonds for Tuesday lunch. In separate jar, soak 1 cup of sunflower seeds for Tuesday breakfast.*

## Tuesday

**Breakfast:** Buckwheat pancakes (1)
Budded sunflower seeds (2)
Fresh fruit in season

Honey, blackstrap molasses or pure maple syrup, with butter
Black coffee, tea or skim milk

**Lunch:** Soaked almonds (3)
Apples

Carob cookies (left over from Monday)
Camomile-orange-peel tea or skim milk

**Dinner:** Roast leg of turkey
Gravy
Mashed potatoes (unpeeled)
Banana fruit cake (4) with whipped cream

Buttered carrots
Cranberry-orange, or orange-apple salad with honey
Black coffee, hierba mate tea or skim milk

*Do ahead: Soak 1 cup of lentils for sprouting for Thursday dinner.*

## Wednesday

**Breakfast:** Granola with fresh or dried fruit and milk, cream or fruit juice — Hot whey with or without a teaspoon of molasses

*Do ahead: Soak figs for Thursday breakfast. Freeze bananas for Thursday dinner.* (See recipe "7" this Phase.)

**Lunch:** (left-overs from dinner)
Whole wheat pocket bread filled with chopped turkey, lentil sprouts, mashed potato and tomato — or any grated vegetable or chopped lettuce
Olives
Hot or chilled lemon grass tea

**Dinner:** Millet-vegetable casserole (5)
Honey-butter glazed parsnips (6) or carrots — Cabbage salad
Frozen bananas (7)
Black coffee, cinnamon tea or skim milk

## Thursday

**Breakfast:** 2-minute eggs on whole wheat toast — Dish of figs
Black coffee, tea or skim milk

**Lunch:** Rye crackers (as Wasa Bread or Zwieback) spread with avocado paste (8) — Celery sticks
Pears
Black coffee, shave grass tea or buttermilk

**Dinner:** Lentil soup (No. 2) (9)
Corn stove-top muffins
Strawberry jam (10) — Leaf lettuce salad with sour cream dressing
Hibiscus tea with Vitamin C and honey

## Friday

**Breakfast:** Oatmeal with butter and nuts
Fresh fruit in season — Hot whey drink, black coffee or tea

**Lunch:** Egg sandwich on whole grain bread
Zucchini sticks — Orange and raisins
Hot or chilled bouillon or tomato juice

**Dinner:** Beef stew with potatoes, carrots, onion, celery
Buttered peas — Green salad
Applesauce cake made with whole wheat (11)
Birthday lemon-grass tea with spices added

43

## Saturday

**Breakfast:** Soft scrambled eggs    Orange juice
Barley stove-top muffins (12)    Black coffee, tea or skim
Raisin jam (13)    milk

**Lunch:** Split pea soup    Plate of vegetable sticks and
Rye crackers or Zwieback    avocado
Black coffee, tea or skim
milk

**Dinner:** Rabbit-noodle casserole (14)    Date-butterscotch pie (15)
Sliced tomatoes and    Black coffee, tea, skim milk
cucumbers
Olives, ripe

*Do ahead: Soak 1 cup whole grain oats for sprouts for Tuesday breakfast.*

## Sunday

**Breakfast:** Whole wheat waffles or    Butter
pancakes (Make your    Farmer or white cheddar
favorite recipe with whole    cheese cubes
wheat instead of white    Fresh fruit in season
flour)    Black coffee, tea or skim
Molasses, sorghum or rice    milk
syrup

**Dinner:** (Mid day)    Whole wheat rolls
Roast lamb or roast beef (16)    Fresh or frozen berries,
Baked sweet potatoes    sweetened if necessary
Buttered cauliflower    with date sugar and
Green salad    garnished with a dollop of
whipped cream sweetened
with honey
Black coffee, tea or skim
milk

**Supper:** Brown beef or lamb soup (17)    Cabbage-pineapple salad
Papaya seed pepper (18)    Hot or chilled chocarob
Fig jam
Barley stove-top muffins

Hurrah! You have just eaten through a week of foods containing no white flour, *cause célèbre* for rejoicing. Refined white flour has only 15% of the nutrition of whole wheat! As though that weren't insult enough, white flour is bleached with chlorine which destroys more of the few remaining B vitamins. Small wonder that atherosclerosis was *unknown* before 1910, when bleached white flour came into general use. Pastries, pies, cakes and delicate, doughy (and tasteless) white bread rose in production to heroic proportions after 1910. As these rose, so did the consumption of refined, white table sugar. The public increased its intake of white-flour-sugar products to nearly four hundred percent from 1910 to 1970!

If, in testing yourselves for food allergies, you have found that someone of your family is allergic to wheat, you can turn to buckwheat (a vegetable seed, not a cereal grain), rice, millet, the root vegetables, carob, etc., for good starch sources. (Details on allergies are contained in Part II.)

We congratulate those of you who have had the desire and self-discipline to carry on your diet change to this point. Be thankful and celebrate! You've passed a real milestone. Know that you are accomplishing what many would like to do. Count your blessings and proceed.

## Exercises for Phase III

The exercises in this Phase are different. They are for better muscle tone where it is needed and good breathing habits. They also can stabilize weight. The overweight can lose pounds, the underweight can gain, and the just-rights maintain their status quo.

Open the window or door, or exercise out-of-doors.

1. Lie flat on the floor, or padded deck or ground, feet straight out in front, arms to the sides. As you inhale, slowly bring the arms straight up over the head to the floor. Exhale as you bring them down to your sides again. Do this three times.

2. Slowly, to a steady count of ten, lift the legs to straight over your hips, then exhaling, let them down to a steady count of ten. You may need to grasp the leg of a heavy piece of furniture to help you, but don't worry. With practice you'll be able to do the exercise unaided. According to Dr. Dittman, a back therapist, this is the most effective exercise for strengthening the lower back.

3. To do this exercise, you may need to put your toes under a heavy, low piece of furniture like a dresser or sofa to hold your feet down. Now, lying flat with arms on the floor over the head, start raising your arms, then the head and shoulders, slowly rolling forward to a sit-up position. Sit straight, pushing the crown of the head up for a steady count of ten, then slowly lie back down, keeping the feet on the floor, and extending the hands and arms over the head, to a count of ten to flat on the floor. Relax.

This exercise and Exercise #2 of this Phase strengthen stomach, back and leg muscles. It is strenuous. Do only once the first day if you are overweight or new at exercising. Do not repeat more than three times. Increase only a time or two each day during the week to seven or ten times. This is a great muscle toner if you progress comfortably and avoid overdoing.

## Recipes for Phase III

### 1. BUCKWHEAT PANCAKES
### (Similar to Stove-top Muffins)

2 C. buckwheat flour

3 t. baking powder

1 t. S. A. plus ¼ t. salt, or ½ t. salt

1 egg

3 T. oil

2 C. water

Mix flour, baking powder and S.A.-salt in large bowl. In a hole made in the flour, add egg, oil and 1½ C. water, stirring until all lumps are gone. Add the rest of the water. Bake on a grill or skillet, and serve.

### 2. BUDDED SUNFLOWER SEEDS

1 C. sunflower seeds

2 C. water

Put the seeds in a pint jar and cover with net or sprouting lid. Wash and drain, then add the 2 C. of water, setting aside for the night. Next morning drain, saving the soak water to drink, put in soup, etc. (it's full of minerals). Wash and drain. Buds are ready to be served or refrigerated. They keep 2 to 3 days.

### 3. SOAKED ALMONDS

½ C. almonds

1 C. water

In small jar, put almonds and water and allow to soak from 4 to 12 hours at room temperature.

Drain, putting soak water, rich in minerals, on soil-growing plants, and wash. Serve or store in refrigerator without a lid. They will keep several days. Soaked nuts of any kind are easier to chew and digest than unsoaked ones.

## 4. BANANA FRUIT CAKE

1½ C. whole wheat pastry flour

1½ t. S. A. or ½ t. salt

½ t. cinnamon (optional)

¾ C. chopped sunflower seeds

¾ C. raisins

½ C. chopped nuts

¼ C. oil

2 eggs

½ t. vanilla

1 C. mashed bananas

1 to 2 T. honey

Mix dry ingredients. In separate bowl, mix raisins and nuts with 2 heaping t. of flour mixture until all particles are coated. To this add oil, eggs, vanilla, bananas and honey. Stir in the flour and 2 or 3 T. of water. The batter should be quite stiff. If too stiff to stir well (there may be a difference in dryness of the fruits), add another T. or so of water. Bake in 9-inch square pan at 350° for 30-35 minutes, or until lightly browned. Serve with or without whipped cream.

## 5. MILLET VEGETABLE CASSEROLE

1 C. millet

2 C. boiling water

1 t. S. A. and ½ t. salt

1 or 2 T. butter

½ C. fresh or frozen peas

½ C. carrots, fine-grated

1 T. chopped onion (optional)

Pour the water over millet, S. A. and salt, bring to a boil, then simmer for 30 minutes and set aside. When slightly cooled, add peas, carrots and onion, and fold into the millet being careful to keep it fluffy. Serve in pre-heated dish. This is a favorite dish in our family. We all enjoy the sweet, full flavor of the raw, crunchy vegetable bits.

# 6. HONEY-GLAZED PARSNIPS OR CARROTS

4 to 6 large parsnips or carrots

1 to 2 T. butter

¼ C. steam water

¼ t. salt or 1 t. S.A.

1½ T. honey or molasses or 2 T. barley malt syrup

½ C. sesame seeds

Steam the parsnips or carrots until tender. If parsnips are more than 1½ inches in diameter, cut in half lengthwise. In separate pan, melt butter and honey, molasses or barley malt syrup and ¼ C. steam water over a pan of hot water, stirring well. Pour immediately over parsnips or carrots, sprinkle sesame seeds over the top, and serve.

# 7. FROZEN BANANAS

6 to 8 very ripe bananas (turning black but not bruised)

Peel bananas, seal in a plastic bag and freeze. When frozen, remove from bag, slice into chilled dishes and serve immediately for very sweet, exciting dessert.

# 8. AVOCADO PASTE

1 ripe avocado

Dash of celery powder, dill weed, onion and/or garlic powder (optional) or your favorite seasonings

1 T. apple cider vinegar or lemon juice

2 t. tamari sauce

¼ t. salt or 1 t. S.A.

Peel and mash avocado to a smooth cream. Add the rest of the ingredients in the order given, and mix. Serve on crackers, toast or bread sticks. If your taste, like ours, goes for mild flavors, mix only vinegar or lemon juice and a dash of salt and enjoy the rich buttery taste of the avocado on rye crackers.

# 9. LENTIL SOUP (No. 2)

2 C. sprouted lentils

2½ C. water

Set aside ½ C. sprouted lentils. Boil the rest in the water for 15 to 20 minutes. Add the vegetables

1½ C. fine-chopped
vegetables (celery,
cabbage, zucchini,
tomato, carrot, onion,
etc.)

1½ t. S. A. and ½ salt

1 to 2 T. butter

and cook three minutes, then set
aside to cool slightly. Add the
butter, salt and ½ C. uncooked
lentils and serve at once for a
wonderfully satisfying main
dish.

## 10. STRAWBERRY JAM

1 C. fresh or frozen
strawberries,
unsweetened

½ C. well packed, seeded,
sticky dates, cut up

Mash the fresh or thawed strawberries and, with the separated
date pieces, put in blender. Let
sit 15 or 20 minutes for dates to
soften. Blend to a cream or work
and whip by hand until fruits are
creamy. You may have to add a bit
more water. If it is a thinnish
cream, don't worry. It thickens
when chilled. Serve at once or
chilled.

## 11. APPLE SAUCE CAKE

2 C. whole wheat pastry
flour

3 t. baking powder

½ t. salt or 1 t. S. A. and ¼ t.
salt

½ t. cinnamon

½ t. nutmeg

1 C. warm apple sauce

3 T. oil or butter

2 eggs

¼ t. vanilla

¼ to ½ C. honey

½ C. water

Mix dry ingredients. Add all the
rest in the order given. Stir to a
smooth, thick dough. Bake in 8"
x 11" pan at 350° for 30 or 35
minutes, 40 minutes for pyrex
baking dish. Serve warm and
plain, or with butter, whipped
cream or hard sauce.

*Note: We make this during apple
season with raw apple sauce made in
the blender.*

# 12. BARLEY STOVE-TOP MUFFINS No. 2

(Use the recipe for Corn Stove-Top Muffins, substituting whole barley flour for cornmeal or corn flour.)

# 13. RAISIN JAM

1 C. raisins

½ to ¾ C. warm water

Blend raisins and water until smooth. Or fine-grind raisins, soak in the water, then mash and whip to a jam consistency. Chill and serve.

# 14. RABBIT-NOODLE CASSEROLE

1 young, dressed rabbit (about 1½ lbs.)

¼ lb. whole grain, vegetable or buckwheat noodles

2 C. boiling water

1 t. salt or 1½ t. S.A. and ½ t. salt

1 T. tamari sauce

Boil or slow-bake the rabbit in covered pan until tender. Cool, de-bone and dice. Cook the noodles in 1½ to 2 C. water with the salt and S.A. until tender. Add the rabbit and tamari sauce. *Note: This recipe makes enough for 8. Any left over can be frozen.*

# 15. DATE BUTTERSCOTCH PIE

10 graham crackers (made
with honey)

1½ C. sticky dates, seeded and
chopped

1 C. hot water

2 T. butter

1 T. gelatin

¼ C. cool water

¾ C. boiling water

½ T. almond flavor

½ C. chopped nuts

Roll crackers to make crumbs and line a 9-inch pie plate. Mix dates with hot water and butter. Work to a smooth mass and set aside. Moisten gelatin with cool water, then add the boiling water; stir until dissolved and allow to cool. When these ingredients are cool, mix together the dates with the gelatin, and blend. Or whip by hand until a creamy mass. Pour over graham cracker crumbs, sprinkle with nuts and refrigerate until firm (about 3 hours). Top with plain or honey-sweetened yogurt or whipped cream for a rich, nutritious, sweet dessert with no refined sugar.

# 16. ROAST LAMB OR ROAST BEEF

Braise the roast slightly in an iron skillet, then place in a covered pan for moist roasting in a slow oven. When meat is tender, remove from pan for serving, then pour the light brown liquid in a jar. Cool and refrigerate.

# 17. BROWN ROAST SOUP

Remove the hard fat from the brown stock of Sunday dinner's roast. Add enough water to make a scant quart and bring to a boil. Dice scrubbed, unpeeled potatoes, onion, and celery stalk. Add to broth. Boil 5 minutes, season to taste, and serve.

# 18. PAPAYA SEED PEPPER

Wash papaya seeds, drain, then dehydrate or dry indoors in dry place or in sun. Grind in seed mill for a mild, zesty pepper free from preservatives. Keep refrigerated.

*Note: When we eat an occasional papaya. we wash and freeze the seeds until we have accumulated at least half a cup. then we dry or dehydrate and grind them for pepper.*

# Phase IV

*" . . . Do you not know that your body is a temple of the Holy Spirit who is in you, whom you have from God, and that you are not your own? . . . therefore, glorify God in your body."*

1 Corinthians 6:19,20

In this Phase you reach the half-way point of your progress through the transitional program, yet psychologically you are much farther ahead. You have already gotten into the *swing* of change. Each new alteration in your diet becomes progressively easier. You will scarcely miss what foods have been left out of this week of menus.

So anticipate! Enjoy! Know, through trust and inspiration, you are truly succeeding in turning your way of living toward health, strength, faith and contentment.

## Special Foods Shopping List

Brazil nuts
Tahini (Sesame seed butter)

Popcorn
Whole buckwheat grains (hulled)

Granola (with honey)

## Daily Menus

### Monday

**Breakfast:** Millet stove-top muffins (1) with soft poached eggs

Grapes
Black coffee or tea

*Do ahead: Soak 1 cup sunflower seeds for dinner. Wash and soak 1 C. brown beans in 2 C. water for Monday dinner.*

**Lunch:** Bananas
Brazil nuts

Carob tea with a dollop of butter or cream

**Dinner:** Brown beans (2)
Rye bread or Zwieback or Wasa crackers
Sesame seed cheese (3) spread or Tahini (the latter at co-op and health food stores)

Spinach-zucchini-celery salad
Raw applesauce (4) or whole apples
Black coffee or tea

*Do ahead: Soak prunes in lukewarm water for Tuesday breakfast.*

## Tuesday

**Breakfast:** Rolled oat cereal with    Soaked prunes
butter, barley malt syrup    Black coffee, tea, water or
and coconut    fruit juice

**Lunch:** Whole wheat,    Sunflower seed buds
avocado-cucumber    (sprouts)
sandwiches    Tomato juice

**Dinner:** Baked white fish    Carrot salad
Lemon-butter white sauce    Orange slices with coconut
Steamed turnips    Black coffee or lemon-grass
tea

## Wednesday

**Breakfast:** Granola served on top of a    Black coffee or tea
bowl of sliced bananas
afloat in pineapple juice,
or apple, prune or orange

*Do ahead: Soak 1 C. buckwheat overnight. Wash and drain morning, noon and night until sprouts are ⅛ to ¼ inch long. Spread on large tray to dry in sun or over stove pilot light (place small foil pan to deflect heat and prop up 2 inches over them) or turn oven to 200°, then turn off and put in the tray of buckwheat, or dry in a dehydrator.*

**Lunch:** Almond butter on rice cakes    Hot or chilled hibiscus tea
Carrot sticks    with lemon and honey

**Dinner:** Brown rice casserole (5)    Carob pudding (6)
celery sticks    Black coffee, camomile tea or
water

## Thursday

**Breakfast:** Corn meal mush with butter    Grapefruit or oranges
and nut meats (7)    Black coffee, tea or carob
drink

*Do ahead: Soak 1 C. navy beans to be cooked for dinner.*

**Lunch:** Chicken-rye sandwich with    Oatmeal-raisin cookies (Use
alfalfa sprouts    any oatmeal cookie recipe,
Cherry tomatoes    substituting water for
Coffee, mint tea    milk, whole wheat flour
for white, honey for
sugar.)

**Dinner:** Navy beans with grated carrots, celery
Buckwheat stove-top muffins

Date-berry jam
Fruit salad (raw)
Black coffee, camomile tea

*Do ahead: Soak pumpkin seeds for sprout buds for Saturday breakfast. Soak sunflower seeds for budding for Friday. Marinate slices of tofu in pure, aged soy sauce for Friday lunch.*

## Friday

**Breakfast:** Soft scrambled eggs (8)
Whole wheat or multi-grain bread toast

Fresh fruit in season
Alfalfa leaf tea or black coffee

**Lunch:** Whole wheat (or multi-grain) sandwich of butter, marinated tofu and romaine leaves

Brazil nuts
Apple
Rosemary tea

**Dinner:** Vegetable plate (9)
Sunflower seed buds in butter (10)

Pecan pie (11)
Cinnamon tea

*Do ahead: Soak ¾ C. barley in 2 C. water for hearty Saturday soup.*

## Saturday

**Breakfast:** Hot chocarob
Rye-raisin muffins (12)

Grapes or fresh fruit in season

*Note: Don't be shocked that barley and rice are served one after the other. It is part of the transitional plan to a rotation diet in which you repeat foods no oftener than every fourth day.*

**Lunch:** Barley-vegetable soup (13) with floating tofu cubes
Rice bran stove-top muffins (14)
Dates

Vegetable sticks (carrot, jícama, zucchini, crookneck squash)
Clover-licorice tea

**Dinner:** Meat loaf (15)
Baked potato
Green beans

Green salad
Applesauce cake
Shave-grass or lemon-grass tea

*Do ahead: Soak almonds overnight for Sunday supper; drain and refrigerate.*

## Sunday

**Breakfast:** Whole wheat waffles or
                pancakes with honey

Fresh fruit in season
Mint tea or black coffee

    *Note: For super nutrition and a taste thrill, mix 2 T. of flaxseed meal and ¼ C. warm water in ¾ C. honey and serve over waffles or pancakes.*

**Dinner:** Baked or poached fish
           Brown rice
           Chinese vegetables

Tomato
Carob chips and raisins
Hierba mate tea

**Supper:** Soaked almonds
           Platter of fresh fruit

Popcorn or buckwheat
    crunchies (16)
Sassafras tea with honey

Voilà! There! If all went well, you just had a week of no milk or milk products except butter, which is a balance between hard and soft fats. Butter contains natural vitamin D, necessary for the assimilation and distribution of calcium. All cells need calcium. Allergists say that dairy products, except butter, cause problems of one kind or another to over half of the people in the United States, including children. Maybe that's why God did not include milk in His diet instructions for mankind. Or maybe it was because milk is necessary for only the very young.

Anyway, we don't need milk, and we soon learn not to miss it and not to care for it. So for that half of the family that can't handle milk, there's now a way to avoid it without taste or nutritional sacrifices. Since heavy cream is mainly butter fat, it can be used by most people.

There's more later on milk and how it can cause such illnesses as asthma, colitis, cataracts, sinus trouble, etc.

For now, carry on. We know it isn't always easy. But before long you'll see that you are spending less money for food, less time in the kitchen "un" cooking, even less time cleaning up! And it will get better as you eliminate more health suppressing costly foods that take longer to prepare and clean up after.

So sing a song of praise and be glad. You are well on your way with even more joy to come!

# Exercises for Phase IV

1. Stand with feet fifteen to twenty inches apart. With hands on hips, bend down as far as is comfortably possible, then slowly move the torso to the left as far as is comfortable, then on around to leaning back with head tilted back as far as possible. Continue on the right as far as possible without straining, then return to the original bent-over position. Continue on another slow, giant torso swing two more times,

then stand up straight and relax in position for a few moments, arms hanging limply.

2. Still standing with feet fifteen to twenty inches apart, extend the right hand up and the left hand down. Now slowly bring the right hand down in a giant swing, to touch the left toe while the left hand, stretched out in the opposite direction, is extended up and back of the torso a little. The left hand continues in its giant up-position swing and slowly descends in an arc to touch the right toe as the right hand swings in a circular motion to extend above and slightly back of the torso. This is called The Windmill, and is a refreshing stretch exercise. Accompany the exercise with a deep exhale as one hand goes down to touch a toe and inhale as the other hand goes to touch the other toe. Do the complete windmill 2 or 3 times at first, increasing a time or two each succeeding day.

3. Stand with feet six or eight inches apart, head pushed up at the crown. This makes you stand tall. Extend the arms straight out from the sides, level with the shoulders, fingers extended. Then spring the arms back, *one. two. three.* as far as possible without strain. This stretches the muscles across the chest and shoulders, those muscles that suffer most neglect since most of our daily work is done with our bodies slightly stooped over—housework, child care, most manual labor and office work. This is a good stretch exercise to do a few times before going to bed to help you relax and fall asleep more readily.

# Recipes for Phase IV

## 1. MILLET STOVE-TOP MUFFINS

These muffins are made exactly like Corn Stove-Top Muffins. For serving with poached eggs, however, we do something different. We bake them on skillet or griddle in doughnut circles and serve on pre-heated plates with the eggs in the hole. A family delight!

# 2. BROWN BEANS

1 C. brown beans (2 C.
when soaked)

2 C. water

½ bell pepper and/or
medium onion,
fine-chopped

½ t. salt and 1½ t. S. A., or ¾
t. salt

½ t. celery seed or celery
powder

¼ C. sour cream or 2 T.
butter

Soak beans 8 to 10 hours. Slow-cook in soak water 1 hour or until tender. (Soaked or sprouted beans will not mush up when cooked like cooked dry beans.) Add bell pepper, onion, and celery powder and cook 5 minutes. Remove from heat and let cool slightly, then add the S.A.-salt and the sour cream or butter. Serve as a main dish or add hot water, vegetable stock or sunflower seed or buckwheat soak water and serve as a soup for a main course.

# 3. SESAME SEED SPREAD

2 C. sesame seed meal made
with fine-grind food
chopper or processor or
seed mill

2 to 4 T. oil or water

½ t. S.A.

*Note: Seeds frozen grind better and don't "gum up" in the grinder or mill.*

Mix sesame seed meal, slightly warmed oil or water and S.A. well. At first you may think there is not enough oil or liquid to make a paste. But with the natural oil of the seeds, the paste will emerge. The taste is full-flavored and one you may have to accustom yourself to. At first some like to season with garlic, dill or caraway seed. Eventually you'll probably like it plain, and really anticipate it.

# 4. RAW APPLESAUCE

4 to 6 apples

¾ to 1 C. apple juice or any
unsweetened fruit juice

1 T. honey

Soap-wash, rinse well and slice apples into blender. Add juice (or water) and honey and blend. Or chop and grind apples, add ½ to ¾ C. juice, honey, and mix. Chill and serve.

*Note: If using water and more flavor is needed. add ½ t. ascorbic acid (vitamin C) and 2 T. honey. This keeps the pure. delicate flavor of the apples.*

# 5. BROWN RICE CASSEROLE

1 C. brown rice

2 C. boiling water

½ C. fresh or frozen peas

½ C. fresh or frozen corn

1 t. S. A. and ½ t. salt, or ¾ t. salt

1 T. butter

Wash, drain and simmer rice and water in tightly lidded pan for 20 to 30 minutes. Put peas and corn in double boiler or small pan set in hot water. When warm, add them and butter to rice, tossing to keep rice fluffy. Serve at once.

# 6. CAROBAN PUDDING

4 large bananas

⅛ t. S. A.

1 C. carob powder

2 t. molasses (blackstrap)

½ t. vanilla

Mash bananas in bowl, sprinkle on the S.A. and the carob. Dribble molasses and vanilla over all and, with a fork, work into the bananas for the smoothest, chocolatish pudding ever. Chill and serve.

# 7. CORNMEAL MUSH-WITH-A-FLAIR

1 C. yellow cornmeal

1 C. warm water

1 C. boiling water

1 t. S. A. and ½ t. salt

2 T. butter

½ C. pumpkin seeds

Moisten cornmeal with warm water. Add boiling water gradually, stirring until smooth. Bring to a boil, turn heat to simmer, cover pan and cook 20 minutes. Set aside to cool slightly. Add butter, S.A., salt and seeds. Serve at once.

*Note: For a richer main dish mush, rapidly stir an egg into the mush immediately after it is cooked. Salt to taste.*

# 8. SOFT-SCRAMBLED EGGS

6 or 8 eggs

4 or 6 t. water

½ t. S.A., ½ t. salt

1 T. tamari sauce

Slightly warm your skillet while you break eggs in a bowl and add water, salt and tamari sauce. Lightly grease skillet with butter and pour in the egg mixture, unbeaten. Scramble with a small pancake turner, with burner on low heat. Remove from stove and serve on pre-heated platter while eggs are still shiny-moist.

# 9. VEGETABLE PLATE

2 potatoes

10 broccoli sprigs

8 baby beets

1 C. grated carrot

1 avocado

½ t. S.A. and ½ t. salt

1 T. vinegar or lemon juice

3 T. water

1 pinch garlic or onion powder

In separate pans, steam slightly the unpeeled and quartered potatoes, broccoli, and beets. Separately grate cabbage and carrots. Cream or blend avocado with S.A., salt, vinegar, water and onion and/or garlic (both optional) and put in a sauce bowl. Serve the steamed vegetables on a pre-heated platter and the cabbage and carrots on a chilled one. Serve avocado mixture as a sauce for the cooked and the raw vegetables. A surprise-thrill for all concerned!

# 10. BUDDED, BUTTERED SEEDS

2 C. budded sunflower seeds

2 t. butter

¼ t. S.A., ¼ t. salt

Place the budded seeds in small pan and set in hot water. Add butter, S.A. and salt and stir when butter is melted. Set in pre-warmed custard cups for a superior tasting, complete protein dish. Everyone loves buttered seeds!

# 11. PECAN PIE

8 graham crackers sweetened with honey

5 or 6 ripe (freckled) bananas

1 T. barley malt syrup or 2 t. honey

¼ t. vanilla

⅛ t. almond extract

2 graham crackers

¾ C. pecans

Line a pie plate with crumbled graham crackers. Separately mash bananas, add barley malt syrup or honey, vanilla and almond extract. Mix to a smooth cream, add the fine crumbs of the two crackers and mix, then pour this over the graham cracker lined pie plate. Arrange the pecans over the top. Serve when well chilled.

# 12. RAISIN-BRAN MUFFINS

2 C. rye flour

3 t. baking powder

1 t. S.A. and ½ t. salt

1 egg

3 T. oil

½ C. raisins

¼ t. almond extract

1½ C. water

1 t. molasses

Mix dry ingredients and add the rest in order given. When thoroughly mixed, drop in oiled or lined muffin pans or oiled 9" x 9" baking pan and bake at 375° for 25 minutes for muffin pans or 30 minutes if baked in the 9" x 9". Muffins will be slightly brown and starting to pull away from the pan. Serve at once. *Note: The texture of these muffins is fine but heavy and chewy.*

# 13. BARLEY-VEGETABLE SOUP

¾ C. soaked barley and soak
   water

2 C. finely chopped soup
   vegetables (whatever you
   like and have on hand)

Salt-S.A. to taste

2 T. butter

Bring barley and water to a boil,
cover the pan and simmer 1½
hours. Add the chopped vegetables and cook five minutes. Season to taste, add butter, and
serve.

*Note: Cook only half the vegetables,
adding the rest after the soup has
cooled slightly. You'll have more nutrition and better taste. This is a good
way to gradually get more raw foods
into the diet.*

# 14. RICE BRAN STOVE-TOP MUFFINS

1 C. rice flour

1 C. rice bran

3 t. baking powder

1½ t. S.A. or ½ t. salt

1 T. honey

1 egg

3 T. oil

1¾ C. water

Mix dry ingredients, then the
rest in order given. Stir until
smooth and bake in 3-inch muffins on griddle or skillet. Serve
hot.
*Note: We call these our vitamin B
buns. They are chock full of them,
especially $B_1$. You'll notice extra
energy!*

# 15. MEAT LOAF

1 lb. lean ground beef

1 egg

4 T. oatmeal

½ bell pepper

1 stalk celery and/or 1 onion

1 t. salt

½ t. thyme

Dash cayenne

Chop bell pepper, celery and onion. Mix all ingredients with your hand. Form into a loaf and bake at 325°, partially covered, for 50 minutes. Serve on platter and slice at table.

# 16. BUTTERED BUCKWHEAT CRUNCHIES

1 C. sprouted, dehydrated buckwheat

1 T. butter

½ t. salt

Melt butter over hot water and pour on slightly warmed (over hot water) buckwheat. Stir well. Sprinkle with salt and serve as you would popcorn, which it closely resembles.

*Note: I keep a good supply of sprouted, dehydrated buckwheat crunchies on hand at all times. If buttered, they have to be refrigerated. Buttered or plain, they have dozens of uses—as croutons, over fruit, over ice cream, as pie crust, as soup crackers, etc., etc. And we make crunchie balls of molasses, just as we make popcorn balls.*

# Phase V

*"He who is generous will be blessed. for he gives some of his food to the poor."*

Proverbs 22:9

Think of all the new and different foods and recipes you've now added to your diet! In the next Phase, you'll be adding several more. As you go through the menus of this Phase day by day, you'll hardly be aware of what a big change is subtly taking place in your program of eating.

You will notice we occasionally ask you to prepare some extra food so you'll have enough for the next day's lunch or a meal a day or two down the line, or for unexpected guests. It will save you time and money.

## Special Foods Shopping List

| | | |
|---|---|---|
| Buckwheat flour | Millet | Rosehips tea |
| Pocket bread (whole wheat) | Barley flour | Garbanzos |
| | Sassafras tea | Flaxseed |

## Daily Menus

### Monday

**Breakfast:** 2-minute soft-boiled eggs
Buckwheat muffins

Raisin jam
Rosehips tea with honey or mild black coffee

*Do ahead: Soak ¼ cup garbanzos for budding for Tuesday dinner. Soak 1 cup rye grains for Wednesday breakfast. Wash and drain three times a day after the soak period for the next day or two of sprouting.*

**Lunch:** Whole wheat pocket bread
filled with finely chopped
raw vegetables mixed
with nut butter

Carrot sticks
Dates
Lemonade sweetened with honey

*Do ahead: Soak 2 cups hulled buckwheat in 2 wide-mouth jars for sprouting the next 2 days. To be dehydrated Wednesday for Friday breakfast.*

**Dinner:** Defatted, broiled lamb chops or shoulder cuts
Mashed Potatoes Supreme (1)
Fresh radishes, ripe olives, celery curls
Gravy from browned lamb juices thickened with whole wheat flour
Buttered peas (frozen) (2)
Date Darko Pudding (3)
Spiced herbal tea

## Tuesday

**Breakfast:** Granola with honey
Bananas
Whole wheat toast
Pineapple juice
Mint tea

*Do ahead: Soak almonds for Wednesday breakfast. Refrigerate in fresh water until time to drain and serve. Continue to wash and drain buckwheat 2 or 3 times during day.*

**Lunch:** Chilled Cream-of-Corn Soup (4)
Whole wheat melba toast
Celery stuffed with tahini
Apple
Herbal tea (optional)

**Dinner:** Buttered garbanzos (cooked 20 minutes)
Steamed broccoli
Barley stove-top muffins
Raisins, nuts
Alfalfa-avocado salad
Lemon juice dressing
Hibiscus tea with honey

*Note: If you have not had time to sprout alfalfa or can't get the sprouts at the market, use bibb (butter, Boston) lettuce, finely chopped, instead.*

## Wednesday

**Breakfast:** Sprouted rye cereal (5)
Bananas
Camomile tea

*Do ahead: Continue to wash and drain buckwheat. Sprout 1 cup lentils for Saturday soup.*

**Lunch:** Garbanzo tacos
Celery sticks
Oatmeal cookies
Fruit juice

*Note: For the tacos, mash garbanzos with chopped tomato, onion (optional), bell pepper and alfalfa sprouts and/or shredded spinach.*

**Dinner:** Baked turkey thighs
Millet
Gravy
Beet tops, steamed
Apple-lettuce-raisin salad (6) with butter dressing
Pear cake (7)
Rosehips tea, coffee

*Do ahead: Dehydrate or dry sprouted buckwheat for Friday breakfast.*

## Thursday

**Breakfast:** Barley muffins with date jam   Plate of fresh fruits
Soaked almonds   Hot carob drink, black coffee

*Do ahead: Soak 2 cups prunes. After dinner, refrigerate prunes for Friday's dinner dessert.*

**Lunch:** Turkey rye-bread sandwich   Bell pepper rings
Zucchini sticks   Figs
  Sassafras tea

**Dinner:** Southern spoon bread (8)   Green beans
Raw cauliflower with   Fresh plums
  sunflower seed dip   Lemon grass tea

*Note: If there is Southern Spoon Bread left over, pack in small square mold and store in refrigerator for slicing and serving as butter-fried mush later. Delicious!*

## Friday

**Breakfast:** Soft boiled eggs sprinkled   Whole wheat toast, if
  with buttered buckwheat   desired
  crunchies   Grapefruit
  Clover tea, black coffee

*Note: Buckwheat should be dehydrated by now. Butter some for extra use. Salt to taste. Store dry in sealed jars in cool, dark place.*

**Lunch:** Bananas   Filberts
Hibiscus tea with honey

**Dinner:** Baked fish (prepare more   Baked yams
  than needed for fish   Steamed broccoli
  croquettes later)   Prune parfait (9)
Whole wheat muffins, bread   Hierba mate-mint tea
  or dinner rolls
Cole slaw

## Saturday

**Breakfast:** Barley waffles or pancakes   Soft scrambled eggs
  (use whole wheat recipe)   Fresh fruit in season or
Molasses     bottled apple cider
  Herbal tea or black coffee

**Lunch:** Lentil soup   Raisin-sesame circles (10)
Fried mush   Cinnamon bark tea
Celery sticks

**Dinner:** Lean meat balls in raw tomato sauce (11)

Whole grain noodles or vegetable-whole wheat spaghetti

Olives, ripe or green

Fresh or frozen peas, warm, buttered, raw

Applesauce (raw, made in blender or ground, with peelings, seeds, and 2 t. honey)

## Sunday

**Breakfast:** Buttered oatmeal topped with soft-poached eggs

Fresh fruit in season

Hot licorice tea

**Dinner:** Chicken, dumplings (12)

Buttered corn

Frozen bananas or fresh fruit

Tossed green salad

Sunflower seed dressing

Comfrey-mint tea

**Supper:** Rye crackers (WASA type or Zwieback)

Almond butter (or any nut or seed butter, as sesame seed)

Vegetable sticks

Ripe olives

Licorice tea

Bravo! Great! By following the menus of Phase V, you survived a week of practically no processed foods. Breads, noodles and olives are prepared, but good brands can be found that use no preservatives, stabilizers, chemicals or artificial flavors and color. Health food stores are your best source. The changes in this chapter were slight because with each phase of menus you have been gradually eliminating processed foods.

When we use the term "natural foods," we mean those without additives. They are left in their natural state, whether raw, dehydrated, frozen or cooked.

We are sure, if your appetite is like most of ours, you'll yearn now and then for something like tasty, salted, seasoned, oiled (hydrogenated) crackers-cheeses-fried foods-conventional pies and cakes, and so on. But there is an abundance of delicious, natural starches, cheese and meat-like foods and sweets that you'll enjoy and soon prefer over the conventional junk foods most of us grew up on.

Just hold faith, keep looking up and beyond, knowing there are good days ahead, days without fear of illnesses. To know God and His will is to know inner peace, security and freedom from anxiety.

*Do ahead: Before going on to Phase VI, you should sprout, dehydrate and store two cups each of rye, wheat, oats and buckwheat in order to make new "goodies" that will delightfully take the place of some of the old devitalized things we all used to enjoy and suffer from. Before long your indoor garden will be a part of your kitchen activity, a joy and a blessing to all who partake of your food.*

# Exercise for Phase V

For this Phase we are introducing only one exercise, a yoga type stretch exercise that is relaxing and muscle toning for the torso, arms and legs.

Sit on the floor with feet crossed and back straight. Take a deep breath on a count of seven, inhaling in the diaphragm as much as possible. Hold to a count of ten and exhale slowly, pushing out all air, to a count of twenty.

Now, breathing naturally, deeply, extend the right leg a little to the right of your body. With hands stretched high over the head, start bringing them down slowly toward the extended leg and grasp the leg as far down toward the foot as possible, with head bent over.

You will feel a comfortable pull on the back muscles. Don't be disturbed if you can reach only to your knees or just below. We don't all have flexible backs.

Now, still grasping the legs with your hands, extend your elbows out a little. This will stretch not only longitudinal muscles of the back, but the latitudinal ones as well. Stretch as far as is comfortable. *Do not over-stretch.* Now, hold this bent-over, comfortable position for a count of twenty-one, then slowly rise up to a sitting position with legs crossed, back straight and hands on knees.

Repeat this exercise on the left side, first extending the left leg, etc.

You must always move slowly and stretch only as far as is comfortable. Never over-stretch or hold the position to the point of fatigue. Each day hold this postion ten counts longer until you reach a stretch-holding count of one hundred.

# Recipes for Phase V

## 1. MASHED POTATOES SUPREME

1 to 4 potatoes

1 C. water

1 t. S.A. and ½ t. salt

1 to 2 T. butter

Scrub and boil potatoes (halving if large) until tender. Do not peel. Mash in the cook water. Add salt and butter and whip, and serve.

*Note: Your family may be shocked at peelings left on the potatoes. Remind them that commercial potato chips have their peelings left on and many restaurants serve shoestring potatoes with peelings. By eating the peelings and the cook water, we get most of the potato's abundance of minerals and vitamins. When you throw these away, you feed your garbage can or kitchen sink better than yourself!*

## 2. BUTTERED PEAS, FRESH OR FROZEN

2 C. frozen peas

Pinch of salt

1 T. butter

Place peas, salt and butter in double boiler or pan over hot water and leave until peas are 110°. (You can barely stir them with your finger.) Serve in pre-heated dish. They are super delicious and nutritious.

## 3. DATE DARKO

1 C. seeded, chopped sticky dates

½ C. unsweetened fruit juice

½ C. warm water

¼ C. chopped nuts or sesame seeds

Blend, or mix and whip, until smooth. Top with unsweetened whipped cream and sesame seeds.

## 4. CHILLED CREAM-OF-CORN SOUP

1 lb. package frozen corn

3 C. warm water

1 t. S. A. and ½ t. salt

Place water in blender bowl, then add corn and salt, blend and serve for an original, elegant, fit-for-a-king soup.

# 5. SPROUTED RYE CEREAL

2 C. sprouted rye

2 C. hot water (not boiling)

2 T. barley malt syrup

4 T. unsweetened coconut

¾ C. raisins

1½ T. butter

Salt to taste

Into the hot water put the barley malt syrup, coconut, raisins, butter, salt and rye. Stir and serve in pre-heated heavy soup cups. Or blend the coconut, rye, butter and salt with the water, adding more if needed, add the raisins and serve for a porridge-type cereal. We like it both ways!

# 6. FRUIT SALAD DRESSING

2 T. safflower oil

1 T. molasses

1 T. lemon juice

2 T. water

⅛ t. cinnamon or mace

Pinch of ginger (optional)

Shake all ingredients in a tightly topped jar or bottle. Dribble over salad.

# 7. PEAR CAKE

*Note: This cake can be made with whole wheat, whole rye, or whole barley as well as rice flour.*

1 C. rice flour

1 C. rice bran

½ t. baking soda

1½ t. baking powder

1½ t. S. A. and ½ t. salt

1 T. molasses

2 eggs

3 T. oil

1 C. pears, raw

½ t. vanilla

½ t. almond extract

Mix the dry ingredients. Chop, grind and/or mash ripe pears. Add the pears and the rest of the ingredients and mix thoroughly. Bake in 9" x 9" pan at 350° until lightly browned and pulling away from pan.
*Note: Oil and flour the pan before pouring batter in. Rice-pear cake is fine-textured and more fragile than other whole grain cakes. Serve warm.*

71

# 8. SOUTHERN SPOON BREAD

1½ C. yellow corn meal

1 C. lukewarm water

1 t. salt

2 C. boiling water

1 C. chopped mushrooms

½ C. celery

¼ C. pumpkin seeds

2 T. butter

Dash cayenne or 1 t. papaya pepper

4 eggs well beaten

Moisten cornmeal in lukewarm water. To the boiling water, add the moistened cornmeal, stirring constantly until it thickens. Turn heat on simmer, cover kettle and cook for five minutes more. Add the other ingredients in order given, stirring in the eggs thoroughly. Bake in a buttered or oiled casserole at 325° for 45 minutes.

*Note: If there is left over spoon bread, pack in a square mold and store in refrigerator for slicing and browning under broiler or in buttered iron skillet and serve as fried mush. Children love it as finger food. Delicious!*

# 9. PRUNE PARFAIT

2 C. seeded, soaked prunes

1 orange

2 T. unsweetened coconut or 2 T. sesame seeds

Whipped cream

Grind or chop prunes and add to peeled, sectioned orange and ½ t. grated orange rind. Blend with soak juice (add extra water if needed) or mash and whip by hand to a thick cream. Add coconut or sesame seeds and mix. Pour into parfait glasses, top with whipped cream and garnish with blossoms of nasturtium, violet, comfrey, African violet, or rose or dandelion petals. Chill and serve.

# 10. RAISIN-SESAME CIRCLES

1 C. sesame seeds

2 C. raisins

Grind sesame in seed mill or twice in fine-grind regular food grinder. Grind raisins. In large bowl, work sesame meal into the raisins by hand, then form in a long "sausage," rolling it back and forth on a bread board floured with one of the following: sesame seed meal, carob powder, rice bran or polish, soy flour or any sprouted, dehydrated grain flour. Cover with cloth and set aside for a few hours. Refrigerate. Slice for serving. These Circles are a universal favorite.

## 11. RAW TOMATO SAUCE

2 medium tomatoes, fresh or frozen

1 T. each of chopped

zucchini

celery

apple

parsley

onion (optional)

2 T. flaxseed meal

1 T. tamari sauce

1 t. papaya seed

½ t. dry mustard

Mash or blend tomatoes, preferably with skins, then the rest of the ingredients. Mix in double boiler or pan of hot (not boiling) water until sauce thickens a bit. Pour over slightly cooled meatballs and serve.

## 12. CHICKEN DUMPLINGS

1 C. whole wheat

1½ t. baking powder

½ t. salt

1 T. oil

1 egg

3 to 4 C. chicken stock

Mix dry ingredients, then add egg and oil and mix. The batter will be very stiff. If more liquid is needed, add a teaspoonful at a time. Drop by walnut-size dumplings, a few at a time, into rapidly boiling chicken broth. Dumplings should not be crowded. Cover with tight lid for 7 to 10 minutes. Cook the rest of the batter in dumplings the same way for a scrumptious old-fashioned dinner.

# Phase VI

*"For many walk . . . whose end is destruction, whose God is their appetite . . . who set their minds on earthly things."*

*Proverbs 3:18,19*

If you don't look ahead, you may not realize at first what is the change in this Phase. Nevertheless, it is so important as to have an entire phase-week to make sure this change is made. You can peek ahead, but I daresay you'll catch onto this one even though the change seems slight. To many adults the transition is actually a major one.

While there are other ways to make this alteration in your mode of living, for many this Phase plan, with menus for each day, has proven to be very effective and quite easy.

## Special Foods Shopping List

| | | |
|---|---|---|
| Ginseng tea | Filberts | Honey-sweetened |
| Spearmint tea | Cornsilk tea | granola |

## Daily Menus

### Monday

**Breakfast:** Soft scrambled Mexican eggs (1) or moist Mexican omelet  
Barley or wheat bread toast

Grapefruit  
Hierba mate tea

*Note: Recipe for barley bread in Part III, Transitional Recipes.*

*Do ahead: Soak and sprout 1 C. wheat berries for breakfast Wednesday.*

**Lunch:** Apples  
Filberts and Carob chips

Lemon-grass tea, hot or chilled

**Dinner:** Fish-rice casserole (2)  
Avocado and tomato on lettuce with lemon juice

Buttered beets  
Oatmeal-fig cookies (3)  
Ginseng tea with honey

*Note: Refrigerate remaining fish for Tuesday lunch.*

75

*Do ahead: Soak sunflower seeds for Tuesday dinner. Sprout 1½ C. rye for Saturday granola bars. (To to dehydrated Wednesday.) Soak 1½ C. red kidney or pinto beans for Tuesday dinner.*

## Tuesday

**Breakfast:** Cooked oatmeal with nuts and butter (4)
Licorice tea (naturally sweet)
Fresh fruit in season

**Lunch:** Mock-tuna sandwich (5)
Orange sections with fresh coconut
Cherry tomatoes
Comfrey tea

**Dinner:** Kidney (or pinto) bean soup (6)
Buttered, budded sunflower seeds
Corn stove-top muffins
Celery sticks
Raisin jam
Hibiscus (Jamaica) tea with lemon and honey

## Wednesday

**Breakfast:** Wheat milk (7) (Save hulls; refrigerate)
Granola made with honey (8)
Bananas
Whole wheat toast if desired
Spearmint tea

*Do ahead: Dehydrate or dry rye for Saturday.*

**Lunch:** Romaine tacos (9)
Olives
Pears, fresh or dried
Camomile tea

**Dinner:** Chinese chicken and vegetables (10)
Brown rice
Soy sauce
Carrot cake
Shave grass tea

*Do ahead: Soak 1 C. oats for sprouting for Saturday breakfast.*

## Thursday

**Breakfast:** Soft poached eggs and butter on millet
Fruit in season
Chocarob or Carob tea

*Do ahead: Soak sunflower seeds for budding for Friday breakfast.*

**Lunch:** Peanut butter-date sandwich
Yam or carrot or jícama sticks
Apples
Clover tea

**Dinner:** Beef-noodle stew (11)
Green salad with avocado dressing
Comfrey-mint tea
Fresh or frozen berries topped with honey-sweetened whipped cream, or raisin-sesame bars

*Do ahead: Soak dried apricots for Friday breakfast. Soak ½ C. pumpkin seeds for Saturday breakfast.*

## Friday

**Breakfast:** Cereal topping (12)    Dried apricots
Rosehips tea

**Lunch:** Rye crackers spread with    Grapes
    almond butter    Cinnamon bark tea
Vegetable sticks

**Dinner:** Poached salmon (13)    Whole wheat dinner rolls
Lemon-butter-mustard    Fig jam
    sauce (14)    Fresh fruit slices
Roasting ears or buttered    Lemon grass tea
    corn
Cole slaw

*Do ahead: Soak 1 C. barley for Saturday's soup. Soak sesame seeds for sprouting for Sunday's guacamole dip.*

## Saturday

**Breakfast:** Sprouted oats cereal (15)    Rosehips tea
Pineapple, fresh or dried, or
    juice

*Do ahead: Soak sunflower seeds for Sunday breakfast.*

**Lunch:** Barley vegetable soup    Sliced tomatoes and
Buckwheat stove-top        cucumbers
    muffins    Date cookies
        Cornsilk tea (16)

**Dinner:** Salmon croquettes (17)    Granola bars (18)
Steamed cabbage    Sassafras tea
Caesar salad with avocado
    dressing

## Sunday

**Breakfast:** Fresh fruit plate sprinkled    Applesauce cake
    with budded sunflower    Comfrey-mint tea
    seeds

**Dinner:** Oven baked chicken parts    Barley or whole wheat bread
Baked potato    Frozen bananas
Buttered peas, raw, warm    Hierba mate tea
Spinach-bean sprout salad
    with sesame oil and lemon
    dressing

**Supper:** Plain rye crackers    Plate of vegetable sticks
Guacamole dip (18)    Brazil nuts and dates
Chocarob or carob tea

Salutations! This is a red letter day. You can now join the ranks of all those happy folk who have found the taste adventure of herbal teas is more fun than a conventional coffee or tea break. With dozens of tasty, refreshing teas, there are infinite blends you can experiment with to create your own taste thrills. Such tea condiments as orange or lemon peel—bits of dried fruits such as prunes, pears, peaches, pineapple and so on added to floral teas like camomile or elder flower, red clover or rose petal, provide exciting, energy enhancing, healthful teas. They also make for fascinating conversation. Try it. You'll see.

It takes strength and vision, faith and trust to break away from orthodox living. Not until we make the break, do we realize there is a big, wide world to explore—to thrill to—to enjoy.

You've made the greatest break-away possible, the change of diet, the way we eat. It is the most fundamental fact of life, for without nourishment we perish.

So enjoy, thrill, thanks-give, and praise!

## Exercise for Phase VI

The exercise for Phase VI is another stretch, yoga exercise for relaxation, muscle toning and activation and for digestion.

Sit cross-legged on the floor, hands on knees, back straight. Breathe deeply.

Bring the right foot to the body, knee up. With your hands, place that foot on the outside of the left knee. This will leave the right knee upright. Now, hook your left elbow over the right side of the right knee and, with the left hand and bending over, grasp the ankle. You'll think you can't do this, but persist. You'll eventually succeed. This puts your body in a refreshing twist.

Now with the right hand and arm extended to the right, move it on around toward the back of you, following it with your eyes as far as the arm can comfortably reach back and as far as the eye can still watch it comfortably. Avoid over-stretching.

Hold for a moderate count of twenty-one, then slowly bring the arm, head and eyes back, uncross the left arm and right knee, and sit in the beginning cross-leg position with hands on knees, back straight. Breathe deeply, slowly for a few moments. Then repeat the exercise, bringing up the left knee. Hook the right elbow over the left side of the left knee. Bending over, with the right hand grasp the ankle. Now with the left arm and hand extended to the left, move it on around toward the back of you, watching it with your eye as far as is comfortable. Hold for a count of twenty-one, then slowly return to the cross-leg position.

If we're short of exercise time, we at least do *this* exercise and the one in Phase V. They're restful, rejuvenating exercises.

## Recipes for Phase VI

# 1. MEXICAN SCRAMBLED EGGS OR OMELET

**6 to 8 eggs**

**¼ C. water**

**½ t. salt**

**1 medium chopped tomato**

**1-inch sliver each of fine-chopped onion, bell pepper and celery**

**Dash of cayenne**

Pour all ingredients in an iron or stainless steel skillet, slightly buttered. Set on medium heat. Scramble all as it cooks to a soft, shiny consistency, and serve on warm platter. If making omelet, stir and whip all ingredients together, pour into an oiled omelet pan and bake at 325° about 25 minutes or until the eggs are coagulated but still moist on top. Serve at once.

# 2. FISH-RICE CASSEROLE

**1 C. brown rice**

**2 C. boiling water**

**1 t. salt**

**1½ lb. white fish (boneless)**

**1 T. rounded, whole wheat flour**

**2 T. butter**

**1½ t. S.A.**

**⅛ t. cayenne**

**¼ t. dill weed or seed**

**1 t. lemon juice**

**1 C. fine-chopped mushrooms**

Cook brown rice in boiling water and salt until tender. Steam or poach the fish in ¾ C. water until fish turns an opaque white (a few minutes). Remove fish. Save ⅓ of it for Tuesday lunch. Refrigerate. Now make a paste of the flour and 2 T. water, and thicken the fish broth. Break up the fish into small bits or flakes, add to the rice along with the rest of the ingredients, mixing to retain the fluffiness of the rice as much as possible. Pour into a preheated casserole and serve. Do not cook more. The delicate flavors and the raw mushrooms are a gastronomical delight.

# 3. OATMEAL FIG COOKIES

2 C. oatmeal

½ C. hot water

½ t. salt

2 C. figs (dried)

2 T. honey

1 T. oil

½ t. cinnamon or mace

1 t. vanilla

¼ t. almond extract

Mix salt in water, then add oatmeal to moisten it. Set aside for 20 to 30 minutes. Grind figs and add to oatmeal along with the rest of the ingredients. Mix well to a thick dough. Make into 1½-inch balls, roll in carob or any sprouted grain flour, flatten into cookies and place on cookie sheet. Cover with cloth and allow to season for several hours. Refrigerate for storage.

*Note: These can be warmed or very slightly toasted for serving, or served plain. They are very special either way.*

# 4. OATMEAL SUPREME

2 C. oatmeal

2 C. water (more if a thinner gruel is desired)

1½ t. S. A. and 1 t. salt

½ C. sesame or other seeds

3 T. barley malt syrup or 2 T. honey or molasses

2 T. butter

Cook oatmeal in water and salt until done. Set aside to cool slightly. Add raisins, seeds, sweetener and butter. Serve with fruit juice, or plain, or with milk, whey, or cream if tolerated. Or blend ½ C. coconut in 1 C. warm water, strain and pour over the oatmeal for another supreme treat.

# 5. MOCK-TUNA ON RYE

1 avocado

Fish, cooked on Monday

¼ t. salt or 1 t. S. A.

1 t. vinegar

Your favorite salad seasonings (we like only celery powder)

Mash avocado. Crumble into it the chilled fish, the salad seasonings and vinegar and mix all together. Spread on rye bread and top with another thin, buttered slice, or with lettuce leaves.

# 6. BEAN SOUP-OF-THE-DAY

3 C. soaked beans (kidney or pinto)

2 C. water

1 C. finely chopped or grated vegetables, any or all kinds

2 T. butter

1½ t. S.A. and ½ t. salt

In large kettle, place beans and water and bring to boil, then simmer for 15 to 20 minutes. (Soaked and sprouted beans remain more or less whole when cooked.) Cool slightly. Add the vegetables, butter and salt. Stir and serve in 4 pre-heated cups, reserving a fifth serving to chill for Wednesday lunch.

# 7. WHEAT MILK

2 C. sprouted wheat

3 C. water

2 t. honey (optional)

Blend wheat and water, half of the mixture at a time, and strain for a most pleasant tasting "milk" to be served over granola, other cereals or as a beverage.

# 8. GRANOLA GOLD

2 C. oatmeal

2 C. sprouted, dehydrated buckwheat (buckwheat crunchies)

2 T. fresh wheat germ

½ C. coconut or sunflower seeds or chopped nuts

2 T. butter

1 t. each honey and molasses

1 t. S.A. and ¼ t. salt

Mix the dry ingredients together and set in a warm place 15 or 20 minutes. In a pan set in hot water, melt the butter with molasses and honey and salt. Dribble over granola mixture, stirring vigorously. Chill and serve. Refrigerate for storing.

# 9. ROMAINE TACOS

1 + C. of Tuesday's cooked beans

1 t. chopped parsley

1 T. each chopped alfalfa sprouts, celery and nuts

1 T. buchwheat crunchies

1 t. chopped onion (optional)

Mash the beans and mix in rest of ingredients. Spoon a "sausage roll" of mixture onto a romaine leaf, roll into a taco and secure with toothpicks. Yum!

# 10. CHINESE CHICKEN WITH VEGIES

1 large chicken breast

1 C. water

1 C. cross-cut celery

1 C. broccoli spears

1 C. sliced carrots

½ C. sliced mushrooms

½ C. fresh or frozen peas

½ C. sliced onion (optional)

1½ t. S.A.

1 T. cornstarch

2 T. water

2 T. oil

1 C. sliced jicama, cut in 1" squares or 1 small can water chestnuts, sliced

Bone the chicken breast, cube and put in large, shallow pan with the water. Bring to a boil, then add all the vegetables and salt. Cover with tight lid and boil 4 minutes and no more. Into a smaller pan pour off the liquid (pot liquor) and thicken with cornstarch moistened with water, stirring constantly. Add oil, stirring, then pour over chicken and vegetables. Add jícama or water chestnuts and serve with soy sauce or tamari sauce, and rice.

## 11. BEEF NOODLE STEW

1 lb. beef cubes

2 T. oil or butter

2 C. boiling water

2 C. buckwheat or vegetable noodles

2 C. chopped turnip, carrot, celery and onion (optional)

¼ t. dill seed

Flour beef cubes in whole wheat flour and lightly brown in oil or butter. Add boiling water and simmer until tender (about an hour). Add noodles and cook 10 minutes. Then add vegetables, cook another 5 minutes and serve.

## 12. CEREAL TOPPING

1 C. (about) wheat hulls from Wednesday breakfast

1 C. sprouted sunflower seeds

2 T. melted butter or 4 T. cream

1½ T. honey or molasses or 3 T. barley malt syrup

Pinch salt

Blend. Or mix well. Serve over bananas, peaches or berries to everyone's delight.

## 13. POACHED SALMON

1 fresh salmon of a few pounds or salmon roast

salt

Fit the salmon into a kettle with a tight lid. Cover with lukewarm water. Bring to a full boil, turn off heat and let sit until ready to serve for the most delicious salmon ever. Salt to taste.

## 14. LEMON BUTTER SAUCE FOR SALMON

1 C. of poached salmon water

1 T., rounded, cornstarch or arrowroot

½ lemon, juiced

1 to 2 T. butter

½ t. dry mustard

1 t. S. A. and ¼ t. salt

Measure the poach water into a pan and bring to a boil. Moisten cornstarch or arrowroot, stir into the liquid, and continue stirring until thickened. Remove from heat to cool slightly. Add lemon juice, butter and mustard, and mix. Serve in sauce pitcher with salmon.

## 15. SPROUTED OAT CEREAL
### (A Meal-in-a-bowl)

2 C. sprouted oats

1½ C. hot water

1 C. chopped dates

1 C. budded pumpkin seeds

2 T. barley malt syrup

1 T. butter

½ t. salt

Blend oats and hot water, then stir in rest of ingredients for a porridge cereal similar to cooked. Or mix all ingredients in a pan set in hot water for chewy, super cereal. Serve as is or with wheat or coconut milk, reconstituted whey, milk, cream or fruit juice, as you like it!

## 16. CORNSILK TEA

Save the cornsilk from your fresh summer corn ears and dehydrate or dry for a delicate-tasting, healthful tea. (Good for the kidneys.) Crumble and measure 1 t. per cup of boiling water for tea.

## 17. SALMON CROQUETTES

1½ or 2 C. left-over salmon

2 eggs

3 or 4 T. rice or wheat bran or wheat germ

½ t. papaya seed pepper

½ t. onion powder (optional)

Crumble salmon in a bowl, add the other ingredients and mix. Drop by spoonfuls in an oiled skillet preheated to 350° (Medium). Lightly brown and serve plain, with lemon or with raw tomato sauce.

84

# 18. FRUIT-GRANOLA BARS

1½ C. sprouted rye flour

2 t. baking powder

⅓ t. salt

½ t. cinnamon

½ t. nutmeg

2 eggs

3 T. oil

1 t. vanilla

½ t. almond extract

¾ C. water

1 C. ground or chopped raisins

½ C. chopped nuts

3 T. molasses

1 T. honey

Mix dry ingredients. Into a cup-size hole of the flour, add the rest and mix well. The batter will be stiff. Spread ¼ inch thick in large, flat pan and bake at 350° for 20 minutes. Remove from oven, partially cool, and cut in 1½ by 2½ inch bars and serve Store at room temperature for a few days. (They are so chewy and good they won't last long.)

*Note: When baked. the bars should not pull away from pan. They will appear slightly underdone. This is right. It's what gives them the chewy consistency.*

# 19. GUACAMOLE DIP

1 large or 2 small avocados

1 T. vinegar or lemon juice

2 T. water

2 t. tamari sauce

1 t. powdered dulse

½ t. each of dill weed, dry mustard and onion (optional)

½ C. sesame seed buds

Mash avocado. Add all other ingredients and mix well, or blend. Serve and savor!

# Phase VII

*"My son, eat honey for it is good, yes the honey from the comb is sweet to your taste; know that wisdom is thus to your soul; if you find it, then there will be a future, and your hope will not be cut off."*

Proverbs 24:13,14

Since managing a sprouting schedule ahead of time is necessary, you will need to read ahead before starting Phase VII to see what seeds and grains are required. You will use the sprouts for recipes. At first this may seem a little overwhelming. However, you will soon see that it becomes second nature. You will reach for a jar and sprouting seeds as readily—and much easier and more quickly—as running to the supermarket.

By the time you get through the seventh Phase, especially after the gradual conditioning of the first six Phases, you will be experienced and confident in managing an all-natural, all-raw nutrition program for yourself and your family. The information and practice this seven Phase course provides is invaluable to your own and your family's health.

A few days before starting Phase VII, you will need to sprout 2 cups each of rye, oats, barley or wheat, and buckwheat to make many things.

## Special Foods Shopping List

| Rosemary tea | Cashew nuts | Slippery elm tea |
|---|---|---|

## Daily Menus
### Monday

**Breakfast:** Pumpkin seeds          Watermelon Breakfast-seeds and rind (1)

*Note: Eat pumpkin seeds (same botanical family as the watermelon) first. Then drink the watermelon rind juice which will taste quite sweet, then eat the red meat, all you want, which will taste deliciously sweet. If you don't have a juicer, eat a piece of rind two by four inches. (This invariably becomes a favorite breakfast, giving sustained high energy all forenoon and a feeling of well being.)*

*Do ahead: Soak 1 C. wheat for fermec to make Essene bread Friday. Soak for budding 1 C. sesame seeds for Saturday. Sprout 2 C. (in 2 jars) rye berries for Thursday. Soak for sprouting, 1 C. lentils for Wednesday sprout salad. Soak and sprout 1½ C. whole grain oats for Tuesday.*

**Lunch:** Granola bars (2)        Carrot and celery sticks
Red clover tea (3)

*Note: These bars can be a complete meal. They're excellent pack-and-travel food.*

**Dinner:** Corn soup              Avocado-alfalfa sprout salad
Buttered buckwheat    Raisins and nuts plate
  crunchies, served in sauce Cinnamon bark tea
  dishes or custard cups or
  sprinkled over soup as
  crackers

*Do ahead: Soak 1 C. sunflower seeds for budding for Tuesday. Sprout 2 C. (2 jars) hulled buckwheat for making crackers Thursday and dehydrating for Saturday.*

## Tuesday

**Breakfast:** 1-minute eggs on oatmeal (4)  Grapefruit
Rosemary tea (mild)

**Lunch:** Dates              Sprouted sunflower seeds
Apple juice

*Note: Eat as many dates and "suns" as you want. You'll find you are satisfied before you overeat and will have lots of energy for all afternoon.*

**Dinner:** Nut meat patties (5)     Yam sticks
Yellow squash soup (6)   Zwieback or Wasa type bread
Licorice tea           or buckwheat crunchies

*Do ahead: Soak 1 C. filberts for Wednesday morning breakfast. Soak and sprout 3 C. wheat in 3 jars. On Friday use 1 C. for wheat milk. Refrigerate the two remaining cups to make Essene bread on Saturday.*

## Wednesday

**Breakfast:** Soaked filberts      Apples (all you want)
Chocarob drink or carob tea

**Lunch:** Raw peanut butter, or nut  Carrot sticks
  butter sandwich (7) with Chilled or hot spearmint tea
  chopped dates

**Dinner:** Sprout green salad (8)          Rice crackers with butter
Sesame seed cheese spread (9) Fig jam
Sassafras tea

## Thursday

**Breakfast:** Sprouted rye cereal with          Bananas, sliced on cereal
coconut, raisins, butter,      Comfrey-mint tea
barley malt syrup

*Do ahead: Sprout (bud) sunflower seeds for Friday breakfast.
Make buckwheat crackers. (10)*

**Lunch:** Soaked almonds          Uncooked granola bar
Pears                      Camomile-dried apple (2
slices) tea

**Dinner:** Fresh vegetable stew (11)      Pecans
Ripe olives, cherry tomatoes Jícama sticks
Licorice tea

## Friday

**Breakfast:** Budded sunflower seeds,          Whole wheat toast
buttered, warmed, salted Fresh fruit in season
to taste                   Wheat milk

*Do ahead: Soak unsulfured prunes 10 hours and refrigerate for
Saturday lunch. Soak filberts 10 hours and refrigerate for
Saturday lunch. Make Essene bread (12) for Sunday or refrigerate
wheat and make on Saturday.*

**Lunch:** Cashews                    Vegetable sticks, including
Cabbage wedge                 raw sweet yam (crisp and
Shave grass tea               juicy) for dessert

**Dinner:** Raw pea soup              Rye bread, buttered
Celery sticks             Apple jam (13)
Rosehips tea with honey

## Saturday

**Breakfast:** Cantaloupe—all you want    Pumpkin or squash seeds to
Cantaloupe seed milk shake    supplement the
(14)                       cantaloupe seeds for a high
protein, high energy
breakfast

*Note: Peel the cantaloupe very thin. The greatest concentration of
minerals is in the green layer just under the rind.*

| **Lunch:** | Prunes | Buckwheat crackers |
| | Almonds | Butter or mashed avocado |

*Do ahead: In the blender jar. soak 4 T. flaxseed in 1 C. lukewarm water. Set aside until time to start dinner. then blend. Or grind flaxseed twice and soak in a bowl.*

| **Dinner:** | Meal-in-one salad tossed | Hibiscus tea with lemon or |
| | with flaxseed dressing (15) | ascorbic acid (vitamin C) |
| | Buckwheat crackers | crystals ⅛ t. per C. and 1 |
| | Pecan butter (16) | t. honey per cup |

## Sunday

| **Breakfast:** | 1-minute boiled eggs with | Grapefruit |
| | buckwheat crunchies (17) | Shave grass-mint-lemon |
| | (All you want) | grass tea (equal parts) |

*Note: When you rotate eggs every four days. you can eat several at a time. It has been proven that soft-boiled egg yolks do not cause cholesterol problems. Quite the contrary. they help.*

| **Dinner:** | Cabbage-pineapple salad | Essene bread, warmed and |
| | (18) | buttered |
| | Brazil nut bowl with raisins | Lemon grass tea |

*Note: The salad is the main part of your meal. Eat all you want for a delicious. uncomplicated dinner.*

| **Supper:** | Sesame-sunflower seed dip | Apple and celery plate |
| | (19) | |
| | Slippery elm tea | |

Voilà! C'est accompli! It has been accomplished, the seventh and final Phase. Actually going through the seven Phases of change from a conventional, health suppressing diet to an all-natural, mostly raw, health-giving diet is a major triumph. Cause for much praise! Arriving at and going through the seventh Phase takes the three P's—patience, perseverance and power from on high for self-discipline.

As we pointed out in the introduction, the original instruction for man's eating was given to us through Moses: "*Then God said, 'Behold, I have given you every plant yielding seed that is on the surface of all the earth and every tree which bear fruit yielding seed; it shall be food for you.'*" Genesis 1:29. And His final one: "*And on either side of the river was the tree of life, bearing twelve kinds of fruit, yielding its fruit every month; and the leaves of the tree were for the healing of the nations.*" Revelation 22:2

God's instructions are not a religion. They are a way to eat for an illness-free life. Seed bearing plants mean vegetables and fruits. Vegetables and fruits and their seeds we are to eat. Leaves are for healing according to Ezekiel 47:12

We can eat other things. God does not condemn us for that. The children of Israel were completely healthy so long as they ate God's manna, a form of plant life. They became diseased after, in His permissive will, He allowed them, at their insistence, to go back to eating flesh. They craved the heavily spiced, over-cooked foods of the Egyptians. The same applies to us today. God does not demand that we eat as He instructed. He knows that eating animal flesh results in putrefaction in our bodies which can cause degenerative disease. But he gave us the power of choice. We can choose the way He provided for us to eat—which is the way to have and maintain health—or we can choose to eat according to our will which, in not following God, can lead to illness and disease.

Most people will not go on all raw foods. But most people would have much better health if they ate eighty or ninety percent of their foods raw.

We all have the choice: dead, processed, man-made and industry-tampered foods that suppress health and cause disease ... or living, natural foods for radiant health of body, mind and spirit for the complete person God intended. Which will you choose?

## Exercises for Phase VII

The body alignment, lower back pain alignment exercise of this last Phase is restful, very beneficial and so easy to do.

Lie flat on the floor, hands down at the sides, relaxed. Take a few deep, diaphragm breaths now and all during this stretch exercise.

Leaving the right foot and leg perfectly relaxed, extend the heel of the left foot down as far as possible. Do not raise it off the floor. Hold in this stretching, heel-extended position to a moderate count of seven, then relax it and the leg.

Now, leaving the left leg completely relaxed, extend the heel of the right foot, still flat on the floor, to a count of seven, then relax it. Let the whole body completely relax.

Repeat the heel stretch three times for each leg as you alternate from one to the other. Gradually increase the number of times you repeat the exercise if you feel the need. Three times for each leg is sufficient for many folks.

This exercise sounds so simple it could not possibly be effective. Yet just the opposite is true. We first learned of this therapy for lower back pain from a masseur. Later an osteopathic physician friend told us this therapeutic exercise is the most effective single one for preventing and helping lower back syndrome he has ever found. It's not too much for a sick back or too little for a well one. And it improves body alignment.

## Recipes for Phase VII

## 1. WATERMELON BREAKFAST

Scrub a medium-size watermelon with soap and warm water, rinsing well. Cut in wedges or slices and cut the red meat out of the rind. Juice the rind in a juicer or grind the rind and squeeze out the juice in double nylon net. Serve the juice, then the red meat. Save all seeds, wash in hot water, drain in screen wire colander and store in refrigerator or freezer until you have at least half a cup of watermelon and/or cantaloupe seeds. When you do, add a cup of cantaloupe or melon cubes, ¼ to ½ cup water and blend at high speed until a smooth cream. Strain through screen wire colander for a superb seed milk shake. Serves 2 or 3 people a small glass.

*Note: A famous hotel in Mexico City serves Leche de Melon (Cantaloupe milk) with honey for extra sweetness.*

## 2. GRANOLA BARS (Uncooked)

2 C. sprouted, dehydrated oats, rye, barley, wheat or buckwheat

1½ t. S.A. and ¼ t. salt

½ t. allspice

1 C. raisins

1 C. dates

2 T. oil

1 T. liquid lecithin

1 T. molasses

½ t. vanilla

1 C. fine-chopped or ground nuts or sunflower seeds

Grind sprouted grain to a flour. Put into large mixing bowl, add salt and allspice and mix well.

Separately grind raisins and dates and mix with the remaining ingredients. Add this mixture to the sprouted grain flour mix, cutting it in with a large metal spoon. This part requires the most work. You will think it will never form a dough, but it will. When mixed, work it with your hands to make it all adhere. You might have to lightly sprinkle with water to achieve this.

Press into shallow cookie pan and roll with a glass jar for smoothness. Allow to cure an hour or so. Then cut in

1½" x 2½" bars. Or you can make the dough into sausage rolls and slice after it cures. Store in refrigerator.

# 3. RED CLOVER-FRUIT TEA

4 t. red clover tea

1 dried prune, cut in small bits

2 or 3 bits dried orange peel

4 cups boiling water

1 or 2 cloves

Put all ingredients in a pre-heated tea pot. Pour on boiling water and let sit for 15 minutes. Serve with or without honey.

# 4. EGGS ON OATMEAL

2 C. oatmeal

1¼ C. hot water

1½ t. S.A. and ½ t. salt

6 eggs

2 to 3 T. butter

1 t. papaya seed pepper

Pour water over the oatmeal and salt, cover with lid and set in warm place for oatmeal to moisten.

With pin or sharp pointed knife, put a tiny hole in large end of eggs. Into a pan of rapidly boiling water, place the eggs and boil for 2 minutes. Take from water with large sieve spoon, remove eggs from shell and drop them into the oatmeal. Add pepper and butter, mix well and serve in pre-heated soup cups or cereal dishes. (Our favorite breakfast.)

# 5. NUT MEAT PATTIES

1 C. walnuts (or other nuts), fine-chopped or ground

1 C. each of grated carrots and celery

½ C. fine-chopped cabbage

Dash each of dill weed, oregano, papaya seed or cayenne, onion, etc.

½ t. salt or 1½ t. S.A.

1 to 2 T. flaxseed meal

Mix everything together in order given, using just enough flaxseed to make the mixture adhere after sitting a few minutes. Make into patties and serve. They can be served warm by placing the serving dish over a pan of hot water and topping with pre-heated lid or overturned bowl. These patties are universally liked.

# 6. YELLOW SQUASH SOUP WITH MUSHROOMS

2 6-inch yellow crookneck squash, chopped

1 C. warm water

1 C. chopped mushrooms

½ t. salt

2 T. butter

Pepper to taste

Blend squash, mushrooms and salt with water. Pour into a pan, add butter and pepper and set over hot water. Serve in preheated soup cups.

*Note: This soup can be made with ⅓ C. cream instead of butter. You may need a dash more salt.*

# 7. NUT BUTTER SANDWICH
## (Makes 1)

1 large romaine leaf, doubled, or 2 butter or leaf lettuce leaves

1 C. sunflower seeds

4 to 5 T. water

Salt (optional)

Grind sunflower seeds to a fine meal in grinder or mill. Mix with water to make a stiff butter and spread some on romaine or lettuce leaves. Layer on sliced tomato and cucumber, salt to taste and top with romaine or other lettuce leaves. You'll want seconds!

# 8. SPROUT GARDEN SALAD

1 C. sprouted lentils

1 C. sprouted mung or adzuki beans

2 medium tomatoes

½ cucumber

½ avocado

4 small, fresh radishes and tops or 1 C. watercress or 10 green nasturtium seed pods and a few green leaves

Chop all vegetables and toss with your favorite seasoning and oil and lemon juice or vinegar.

# 9. SESAME SEED CHEESE

2 C. sprouted sesame seeds

4 to 6 T. warm water

¼ t. dry bread yeast

¾ t. S. A. and ⅛ t. salt

Blend sesame seeds with water and yeast to make a thick cream. (It will have a tangy, cheese-like flavor.) Pour in a small, deep dish and allow to age a few hours in a warm place, then refrigerate and serve. It keeps a week to 10 days.

# 10. BUCKWHEAT CRACKERS

3 to 4 C. sprouted buckwheat (2 C. dry measure)

1 to 1½ C. buckwheat soak water

1½ t. S. A. and ½ t. salt

Blend sprouts, water and salt, doing one-half at a time. When a medium cream, spoon 2½-inch circles (1 t.) on plastic or wax paper-lined dehydrating trays or shallow cookie pans. Or pour in a thin sheet on trays or pans. When crackers are almost dry, lift off the trays or pans and carefully turn them over, then peel off the plastic or wax paper. Check the sheet crackers in squares for breaking apart when done, and finish drying. When crisp, cool and store in tightly lidded containers in cool, dry place. Crackers will keep several weeks.

## 11. FRESH VEGETABLE STEW

1 medium potato

2 medium carrots

1 C. green beans, cut

1½ C. water

1 t. salt

1 T. arrowroot or cornstarch

1 to 2 T. butter

½ C. cabbage, chopped

½ C. celery, chopped

1 tomato, diced

1 onion, diced (optional)

1 sprig parsley or mint, fine-chopped

Dice unpeeled potato and carrots, add green beans, water and salt and cook 10 minutes. Pour off the liquid in a small pan and thicken with arrowroot or cornstarch moistened with 2 T. water. Add butter and stir. Add thickening to cooked vegetables, then the rest of the raw vegetables. If the stew has cooled too much, set in a pan of hot water and serve in pre-heated dish.

## 12. ESSENE WHEAT BREAD

*Note: Essene bread can be made with sprouted oats, barley or rye*

4 C. sprouted wheat

1 t. S. A. and ½ t. salt

Spread the sprouted wheat out on large tray for an hour to dry a little. Grind once for coarse, twice for finer textured bread. Mix in the salt and work into 1 large or 2 smaller loaves. Set aside, covered with cheese cloth, in the sun for an hour or two, or in a warm place in the house for 6 to 8 hours. Refrigerate to stop the rapid fermenting action. The bread, different from baked bread, is moist and chewy. It may seem quite strange at first. We suggest you warm it in a buttered skillet on very low heat for a pleasant new taste experience.

There are interesting variations to give the bread more flavor. We season with caraway or dill seed, or add a cup of carrot pulp (from the juicer). Some like onion and/or garlic seasoning. Our favorite, since sprouted wheat is slightly sweet, is to add ½ C. chopped dates to dough for a delicious, tangy sweet bread. Cultivate a taste for Essene bread. It is highly nutritious in quality proteins (amino acids) and carbohydrates (fruit sugars) which are so easy to digest they leave you with abounding energy.

## 13. APPLE JAM

2 medium apples

1 C. dates, pitted and chopped

¼ C. warm water

Core and cut up apples and put in blender. Add dates, then warm water. Blend until smooth and creamy. Put in lidded jam jar, chill and serve. Jam will keep a week to 10 days. If ½ t. ascorbic acid and 1 T. honey are added, it will keep 2 to 4 weeks.

## 14. CANTALOUPE SEED MILK SHAKE

Peel 2 cantaloupes as thin as possible, leaving the green on the cantaloupe. Cut in halves and scoop the seeds and pulp into the blender. Add 2 or 3 slices, cubed. Slice the rest for serving.

With ¼ C. water, blend seeds until a thick, smooth cream, strain through a screen wire sieve and serve in small glassses. We usually add a little water to wash out more of the pulverized seed kernels.

# 15. FLAXSEED DRESSING

4 T. flaxseed soaked in 1 C. warm water

2 T. vinegar

1 T. olive oil

1 T. tamari sauce

Dash cayenne

½ t. celery seed

¼ t. caraway seed

¼ t. sesame seed

1½ t. S. A. and ½ t. salt

⅛ t. onion and/or garlic powder (optional)

Blend all ingredients together, chill and toss with the salad just before serving.

# 16. PECAN BUTTER

1 C. pecans

2 or 3 T. lukewarm water or 2 or 3 T. oil

Freeze pecans, then fine-grind. Add water or oil to make a smooth paste. Chill and serve. Pecan butter made with water lasts a week to 10 days, with oil it will last 3 or 4 weeks.

# 17. EGGS-ON-BUCKWHEAT CRUNCHIES

1 C. Buckwheat Crunchies

2 T. butter

8 eggs

Salt

Warm Crunchies over hot water. Pre-heat heavy soup cups. Boil eggs 2 minutes. Into hot cups put the Crunchies (¼ C. to each soup cup). Remove eggs from shells, dropping 2 in each cup. Add ½ T. butter to each and salt and pepper to taste.

# 18. CABBAGE-PINEAPPLE SALAD

1 medium pineapple,
  peeled

½ medium cabbage, grated
  or chopped

2 medium avocados

2 T. vinegar or lemon juice

2 T. honey (more if
  pineapple is tart)

¼ t. salt

Cut the pineapple in 1-inch pieces, including the heart which is sweet, juicy and a good source of fiber. (Chew it well.) Mash the avocados with the vinegar, honey and salt. Put pineapple, cabbage and avocado mixture, in that order, in a large bowl. Mix, toss and serve.

*Note: This salad seems large but it is correct for four good appetites since it is the main part of the meal.*

# 19. SESAME-SUNFLOWER SEED DIP

1 C. sesame seed meal

1 C. sunflower seed meal

6 to 8 T. water or 8 to 10 T.
  oil

Mix the two seed meals with enough water to make a thick cream. Or mix with oil for a richer, thicker cream. Season to taste. Chill and serve. Any left over dip can be used later, thinned as a salad dressing or as is to spread on zucchini, jícama or Jerusalem artichoke slices.

# Transitional
## Guidelines
### for Your Health

# A Clean Digestive System Is Vital

*" . . . and the leaves of the tree were for the healing of the nation."*

*Revelations 22:2*

No person living for years on the conventional American diet can depend on having a clean, well-functioning, efficient digestive system. People invariably say, "We eat too well for food to be the cause of any illness. Our diet is well balanced. It should give us health." Yes, food *should* give us health. Unfortunately, nutrient-deficient, additive-contaminated food doesn't.

The majority of Americans eat the highly processed, artificially colored, artificially flavored, chemically preserved, devitalized foods offered by supermarkets and restaurants. When they eat a wide variety of conventional processed foods: a wisp of salad, a cooked vegetable, a cooked starch, meat, and a dessert—making sure they get plenty of protein—they feel they have a "well balanced diet." They have followed the dictum of medical orthodoxy for the past fifty years.

Tragically, this diet is not only inadequate but no longer balanced. Since World War II, the American public consumes nearly twice as much beef as before. Nutrition-minded people now realize some of the sad results of eating too much fat-marbled, chemically-contaminated beef. They also realize fried foods and sugary confections cannot compare nutritionally with raw and steamed vegetables and fresh fruits. But no matter how nutritious our food, it will not nourish us if we cannot digest and absorb it properly!

The main barrier to this assimilation process is an unclean gut—a slime-coated small intestine and a putrefactive, mal-formed, mucus-infested, constipated colon. Many therapists—physicians, nutritionists, osteopaths, chiropractors, naturopaths—cite these intestinal conditions as a proven fact and a fundamental cause of most diseases. Environmental toxins and ingested drugs can cause the rest.

Our traditional diet not only does little to cleanse and keep clean our digestive system, it contributes to the problem! For one thing, there is far too little fiber for good digestion and absorption. Processed foods are almost invariably depleted of much of their bulk. White rice, white flour, and many nuts have lost their kernel covering in processing. Such vegetables and fruits as potatoes, carrots and most other root foods, apples, peaches and plums are often peeled, thus robbing us of much essential fiber. Lack of fiber in the diet is not corrected by simply adding wheat bran, an incomplete fiber. Bran is an irritating substance for the gut, causing serious problems in the amount often prescribed for constipation and when taken over an extended period of time. The phytic acid (phytate) blocks the utilization of zinc so essential for iron absorption, for growth in children, especially boys entering puberty, and for metabolizing vitamin B6, magnesium and other nutrients.

We, along with countless others, find psysillium hull (husk) to be a most beneficial fiber to supplement the diet of the person having an elimination problem. It gives a lot of bulk. Without sufficient bulk in the diet to act as a brush for sweeping nutrients along the intestines, foods—especially slow-digesting meats and other animal proteins—putrefy and cooked starches ferment in the diverticuli or the unnatural pockets (ballooned diverticuli) of the intestines. This putrefaction and fermentation is toxic. As such toxins slowly move on and out, they are partially re-absorbed into the blood steam and so give us an unclean system beginning with the bloodstream.

Our liver, the great detoxifier, becomes overworked. When the liver is overworked, the other organs of the digestive system function less efficiently and we see the beginning of degenerative disease which starts in our weakest area or organs. With one person it may be some kind of eruption on the skin, the largest organ of the body. With another it may be the pancreas and adrenals, resulting in hypoglycemia and/or diabetes. With yet another, a toxic system may result in arthritis, eye problems, heart trouble, cancer and so on, ad infinitum.

Obviously, the beginning of recovery from any disease is to clean out the small intestine and the colon, our body's cesspool, and stay on a clean, natural diet. This is true for treating *all* disease.

There are several ways to cleanse the colon, all of them proven effective to one degree or another. We suggest you study each one listed below. (We have tried them all in the last thirteen years since we cleanse at least once a year.) You can choose the one you feel is best suited to your body and mode of living. Or consult your nutrition-practicing doctor: medical, naturopathic, osteopathic, chiropractic or homeopathic.

It is greatly helpful, and may shorten the cleansing time, to take an enema once a day for stimulating the liver, gall bladder and pancreas. We suggest a coffee, tea or vitamin C enema. Take one cup of strong coffee (not decaffeinated) or camomile tea in ¾ quart of lukewarm water, or ½ teaspoon of ascorbic acid powder dissolved in a quart of water. Enemas should be held for up to twenty minutes before expelling. Many find the best place to take an enema is in the bathtub, pre-warmed with hot water, where one can lie down (the best position for enema-taking) and be comfortable with a folded bath towel for a pillow.

1. **Raw Juice Cleansing**—Drink eight or ten ounces of freshly extracted juices from fruits and from vegetables every two or three hours during the day and until retiring. We find fruit makes the best juice to take on arising and vegetable juice the best before retiring. The fruit sugars may be too energizing and tend to keep a person awake. Continue for ten days to three weeks, depending on the duration of digestive problems. Older people, cleansing the colon for the first time, often do better on a three week juice fast. Use only freshly extracted juices. In an emergency, use frozen juices. Herbal teas may be taken during any cleansing program unless otherwise indicated. *(Note: Take 4 ounces of cabbage juice diluted with 4 ounces of water, and 4 ounces of beet juice, tops and root, diluted with 4 ounces of water frequently during the fast.* Follow your raw juice and enema cleanse with a few days of *small* meals consisting of a vegetarian diet of whole fruits, sprouts and vegetables, in that order.

2. **A Watermelon Fast of Three Weeks**—Juice the watermelon rind and drink first, then eat the red meat. Eat as much as you want as often as you want without stuffing yourself. Always save the seeds, washing, draining in a colander and storing in refrigerator for seed and watermelon "shakes" later. Follow with a vegetarian diet of fruits, sprouts and vegetables for at least a few days.

3. **The Lemon-Olive Oil Colon Cleanse**—Into a quart of pure water mix the fresh juice of 4 lemons and 3 or 4 tablespoons of raw honey. On arising take 1 T. of olive oil. Afterwards, every two hours drink a glass of this preparation alternating with a glass of vegetable juice made with at least one fourth part beet, then cabbage juice. Continue for at least three days. Then follow with a fruit diet for a day or two, then sprouts and vegetables.

4. **The Grapefruit Cleanse**—Eat one whole large grapefruit for each meal—breakfast, lunch, dinner—and at bedtime, peeling off only the yellow skin with a sharp knife. Eat all the white with the juicy sections. Eat nothing else. On arising the next day, drink a twelve ounce glass of water and take a camomile tea, coffee or vitamin C enema. Continue for several days on a vegetarian diet.

**5. Water Fast**—Many physicians and therapists prefer a pure water fast. They consider it to be the quickest, most complete cleanse of the colon. A rule of thumb is to fast, taking only pure spring or well water, and perhaps lick a little salt a time or two each day. One should fast until he or she feels well, then continue for several hours or a day to make sure the withdrawal period is over. Enemas help to shorten the time of fasting. A person fasting for the first time should do so under the care of a physician or therapist, or a person well experienced in fasting procedures.

After cleansing, the faster should be kinesiologically tested on each food to determine any allergies. (See next chapter.) Only one food at a meal is advisable for the first few meals. For instance, if bananas, after testing, do not pose a problem, then they can be served, several for the first meal. The faster will notice that his or her stomach will seem to have shrunk, and the appetite is quickly satisfied. This is nature's sign to proceed *slowly* with the taking of food after a fast.

We feel so uplifted, clean, alert, calm and optomistic after any kind of a good cleansing program, that we strive to live regularly on a cleansing diet of all-natural foods. We may break over now and then and eat a conventional food. But after seeing and feeling the body perform something less than optimally, we are once again convinced that the all-natural diet is a super, health-giving, invigorating way of life.

# Discover Your Allergies with Kinesiology

*"Eat thou not the bread of him that hath an evil eye, neither desire thou his dainty meats."*

Proverbs 23:6

The Kinesiology Test for Allergies, or muscle strength test, is coming of age. Discovered and developed by Dr. George Goodheart and further researched by such scientists as John Diamond, M.D., it is being used by physicians, dentists, osteopaths, chiropractors, naturopaths and other therapists. If carefully done, closely following instructions, responsible adults can test each other for food and materials allergies. It is quick. It costs nothing. And, as several physicians have remarked, it is amazingly unerring!

To do the testing, follow these instructions: The subject to be tested stands and extends his or her arm and hand straight out from and level with the shoulder. The person who does the testing (the tester), with one hand on the subject's wrist, pulls down on the extended arm, while the subject resists as much as possible.

Keeping in mind the strength felt in the extended arm, the tester then puts some object like a soft plastic bottle in the subject's left hand. Again the subject extends the right arm and makes it rigid. Again the tester pulls down on the arm. If it is more easily pulled down than in the trial test of strength, the subject is allergic to plastic. His body is weakened by contact with the plastic that is known to be toxic. For maximum strength and freedom from the fatigue factor, he should avoid soft plastics.

A double check can be made on the soft plastic bottle. The subject presses the end of the little finger to the end of the thumb of the left hand with all the strength that can be applied. The tester tries to pull the finger and thumb apart, grasping each at the last joint, thus testing the strength of the subject's hand. Now the tester places the plastic bottle in the right hand while the subject presses together the thumb and little finger of the left. The tester tries to pull the thumb and finger apart. If done so fairly easily (as against pulling them apart with great difficulty

107

before), the subject's body is allergic to soft plastic.

The test was conducted on one patient by another patient in the presence of the doctor who taught us how to do the testing. Here's what the doctor had patients John and Mike do. John was the tester, Mike the subject.

1. Mike extended his right arm straight out from his shoulder, his fist clenched, his arm rigid.

2. John tested the strength of Mike's arm by pulling down on it at the wrist after he said, "Resist me." This showed John how much strength was in Mike's arm. He had to exert considerable effort to pull Mike's arm down.

3. Into Mike's left hand, relaxed at his side, was placed a polyester sock.

4. Mike again made his extended right arm rigid and clenched his fist to resist John's trying to pull it down.

5. John had little trouble pulling Mike's arm down this time. Mike's body was weakened by contact with the polyester, a toxic material. In the present day parlance, Mike was "allergic" to polyester.

To double-check the result of the test, the doctor taught John and Mike the other way to do the same test.

1. Mike pressed the tip of his little finger to the tip of his thumb of his right hand as hard as he could. His empty left hand was relaxed at his side.

2. With difficulty, John pulled the thumb and finger apart. Mike had formidable strength in his fingers.

3. Mike again received the polyester sock in his left hand while he pressed his right finger and thumb together.

4. John pulled Mike's little finger and thumb apart with minimum effort.

5. Again Mike's strength was weakened by contact with polyester.

The doctor gave two small objects to John to do another test on Mike, this time a blind test.

1. Mike extended his arm.

2. John tested the strength in Mike's arm by grasping the wrist and pulling down on it. There was formidable strength in the arm.

3. Into Mike's left hand, held palm up, slightly back of him and out of his sight, John laid the two small objects.

4. Mike again made his arm rigid and clenched his fist to resist John's testing of his strength.

5. John had little trouble pulling Mike's arm down.

The doctor then showed Mike the two vitamin tablets John had laid in Mike's hand, vitamins the doctor thought of prescribing. But with Mike's body showing an allergic response, the doctor, of course, did not prescribe them.

The doctor had John test Mike on kelp tablets, this time using the finger-thumb method. Mike was deficient in several minerals and the doctor wanted not only to know if Mike was allergic to kelp, but how many tablets he should take. He cautioned John to be very careful in assessing Mike's strength before testing the kelp. This test could have been done blind but the doctor chose to have it done open, using the little finger-to-thumb method.

1. Mike pressed his little finger to his thumb (right hand).
2. John had difficulty pulling them apart.
3. John put one kelp tablet in Mike's left hand.
4. Mike again pressed his finger against his thumb.
5. John found the strength in Mike's hand unchanged.
6. John put another kelp tablet in Mike's hand and found the strength in Mike's thumb and finger greater.
7. John put the third tablet in Mike's left hand and found even greater strength in the thumb-pressed-against-finger on the right hand.
8. John put the fourth kelp tablet in Mike's left hand and could hardly pull the thumb and finger of the right hand apart, so great was the strength.
9. John placed the fifth kelp tablet in Mike's left hand and found that the finger-thumb pressure of the right hand was weak.

Thus, according to his "body language message," the proper dosage of kelp for Mike was four tablets (taken with meals).

John did a few more tests on Mike, part of the time using Mike's left arm or hand for the strength testing. (In testing several things at one session, one should alternate the hand and arm used for strength-testing to avoid undue tiring.)

Later at home, the two young men continued the testing at intervals. Mike's favorite vegetables were corn and peas, but he had noticed that he felt sluggish after eating peas. When John did a blind test of the two vegetables by laying a few of first one then the other in Mike's palm, he found that the strength in Mike's hand and arm was greatly diminished when holding the peas.

Mike learned through Kinesiology Testing that he was allergic to peas, peanuts, cooked starches (cereal grains, potatoes, rice), mango, carob, beef, pork, chicken and turkey, plus such over-the-counter drugs as aspirin and Tums, and his favorite brand of toothpaste. He was allergic to scented soap and household cleansers, polyethylene (car upholstery) and synthetic rubber, besides the polyester and soft plastics. By eliminating all those things in his home, he feels great and is over the illnesses he suffered as the result of his many allergies and sensitivities. With his much improved health and diet, he is able to tolerate the everyday toxins he encounters away from home if not exposed to them for too long a time.

Anyone can learn to conduct these tests, provided common sense and a few guidelines are observed. The Kinesiology Test for Allergies is not a parlor game. It is a serious, highly useful test for indicating why the body may be suffering from weakness, dysfunction, fatigue or illness. Here are a few things to keep in mind while testing:

- Do the testing in private, free from distraction.
- Plan to test only a few things at a session.
- Do not continue testing immediately after the subject is found to be allergic to something. The fatigue of the arm or finger-thumb sometimes carries over to another test and affects the results.
- Even though the subject does not test allergic, he or she should not be tested on more than three things in a row because the fatigue in the arm and/or hand may alter the test results.
- Testing is best done by adult members of the family or close friends.
- In testing children, great care must be taken in explaining the rules of the test, then in observing the degree of the strength in the child's hand and arm in both phases of the test.
- In the case of an ill person, test only one thing at a session. The thumb-little-finger test is advisable.
- If the subject tires, he or she should lightly tap three or four times over the thymus gland, about three inches below the center dip in the collar bone, to restore strength.
- If the food or object to be tested cannot be held by the hand of the subject, the hand can be placed against or on top of it.
- Gases can be tested by having the subject breathe fresh air during the preliminary appraisal of the strength of arm and fingers. Afterward, he breathes the gas as the strength of his fingers or arm is tested.

*Note: Both the tester and the subject must remain serious and sober during the testing. Smiling alters results.*

Before anyone can prescribe a proper diet he or she needs to know what foods may cause a problem. If a food causes a sensitivity (allergy), that food becomes a poison that the system has to cope with. If the liver is healthy and can detoxify the unusable food, no particular problem is noted. But if the liver cannot detoxify the offending food, the body has a problem which may show up as indigestion, grogginess, headache, constipation, skin condition, arthritis and so on.

Use the Kinesiology Test carefully to reveal offending foods. The body does not lie. Avoid eating food that cuts the body's energy as indicated by the test. After a few weeks, try eating the food all alone if you do not have full confidence in the Test and see if you feel good after eating it. If not, you know to leave it alone.

About every six months, we retest a food that we were sensitive to. Once in awhile, we find one that no longer gives a problem. In such a case, we eat it only periodically.

In theory, the body should not be sensitive to any foods if it is receiving optimal nutrition. However, in our present society there are many extenuating circumstances that alter our food requirements. There are pollutants that may cause us to need more vitamins. Also, each person on earth may need different amounts of certain nutrients in different combinations. No two of us are alike. The human body is a marvelous, extremely complicated, mechanism. Science does not yet know why some can eat a perfectly good, highly nutritious, pure, natural food and some can't. But the body will tell us if we consult it. Remember that it tells the truth. Follow the rules and use the Kinesiology Test to know that truth.

# How Processed Foods Bankrupt Your Health

*"And His disciples asked Him, saying, Master, who did sin, this man or his parents, that he was born blind? Jesus answered, Neither has this man sinned nor his parents: but that the works of God should be made manifest in Him."*

*John 9:2,3*

How many times have we all heard people say, when serious illness came upon them, "Why did this happen to me?"

Who can answer? Perhaps it is God's way of working his will through us. Perhaps it was a harmful work condition over a period of time. Or the result of an old accident or a genetic condition or birth defect like the blind man's which prompted Jesus to say " . . . that the works of God should be made manifest in us." It may have occurred after years of living on nutrition-lacking, unnatural, tampered-with foods from supermarkets and fast food restaurants. These inevitably lead to the break-down of our bodies and to degenerative diseases. We are not alone. The health of Japan, Canada and Europe—with Asia, South and Central America following close behind—is suffering.

Since we now know the cause of much of our physical problems, we can all do something to prevent our health from deteriorating and to get over diseases! That something is to avoid chemicals in our environment and in our foods, and eat all-natural vegetables, fruits, seeds, grains and animal products.

In Phase I, sugar did not appear. It was the first harmful junk food to go. Why? As every doctor using nutritional therapy knows, and all nutritionists agree, sugar is Public Enemy No. 1!

With sugar out of your diet, you have real cause to rejoice. It is a notorious sleep stealer. Sugar is perhaps the greatest cause of irritability. The high, low yo-yoing of energy set off by sugar leads directly to hypoglycemia, then diabetes. Sugar causes the lion's share of nervous, mental and emotional problems. Sugar triggers hyper-activity in children. It causes teeth to decay. Leaving off sugar means freedom from migraine headaches and the pain of arthritis for countless people. Sugar creates stress in the body that requires many more vitamins than it may receive in a conventional diet. This means deficiencies that lead to sickness. Problems and degenerative diseases resulting from consumption of sugar are legion, causing people to spend billions of dollars a year needlessly.

Historians say that sugar addiction, along with lead poisoning, caused the fall of the Roman Empire. Caesar, the Senate and high government officials often feasted on sweets. Soon after such an indulgence the energy of their poisoned bodies severely dropped, leaving them exhausted, their emotions quarrelsome and irritable, their minds drastically weakened, their power of concentration destroyed, their thoughts negative.

Alexander the Great as a very young man learned how to conquer the then-known world. Before a battle he would send scouts into the enemy camps with plenteous gifts of sugary confections. The morning afterward, he would attack. The enemy, after a rowdy evening "high," suffered the inevitable "low" a few hours later, and had neither the strength nor the will to fight hard enough to be effective. Alexander's army easily routed them.

After sugar comes a number of foods causing ill health, each creating about as much malnutrition as the other. First, there is white flour. Eighty-five percent of the nutrition has been taken out when the processers remove the wheat germ and the bran, then bleach what's left with chlorine, a poison. We give the pigs the oil and vitamin-rich germ, the mineral-and-vitamin-rich bran. They are healthy, active and disease free. We give our families white bread, white crackers, cakes, cookies, pastries and pastas and cause them to be malnourished and easy prey to disease.

Not only are white flour products criminally lacking in nutrition, they are loaded with poisonous chemicals such as artificial colors (the worst, say bio-chemists), artificial flavors and flavor enhancers, deadly amounts of salt and a host of preservatives and artificial ingredients masked as foods. These poisons are so ubiquitous, they affect nearly everyone.

We are a nation of people with such toxic-laden, sick bodies that few are truly healthy. Oh, we function, we produce, we reproduce. Very few, however, feel radiant on arising and go through the day maintaining high energy. Over fifty percent of our children even show signs of deficiencies, allergies, weaknesses. And in the last twenty-five years birth defects and mental retardation have doubled!

How many of us have been diagnosed as having some persistent problem such as athletes foot, varicose veins, dandruff and flaky skin? Or maybe it's gas, splitting peeling fingernails, dry burning lips, headache, late-afternoon and upon-arising tiredness, blurry vision, constipation, diarrhea, arthritis, psoriasis—even cancer. And the doctor consoles us with the words, "We all live with something."

Yes, we all live with something because most of us are, or have been for some extended period, malnourished, overfed (half the population is overweight) and overdosed with drugs, chemicals and indigestible foods. But the marvelous news, the great news, is that when nutrients in a natural, living form with no chemicals present are supplied, health is restored and energy abounds!

Commercial meats, once believed to be so necessary for that restoring of energy and health, no longer do so for us. Animals are shot with stilbesterol for rapid growth and fed antibiotic-treated grains. Before slaughter they may be given tranquilizers and bleeding agents. After slaughter the meat may be injected with chemicals to prevent it from discoloring and to tenderize it.

Most chickens, raised off the ground in cages, are fed an enriched diet and medicines to prevent fungus. They are forced to grow fast and/or to produce eggs. Cancer is epidemic in these commercial establishments. Hens are forced to produce an egg every 32 hours. After a year or two of accelerated laying, the hen's body is too emaciated to be slaughtered for the broiler market. It ends up in a can of soup. Dressed broilers and fryers, prepared for distribution across state lines, are dipped in *formaldehyde* before packaging!

Even fish, once the purest of all, are often formaldehyde-treated if the fishing boats are out for a few days, despite the fact that the fish are kept on ice.

Cereals and crackers, snack chips and bits are heated to over five hundred degrees to make them keep forever on the shelf. Vitamins, enzymes, starch, fats and even some minerals are destroyed! They are converted to garbage for our poor, undernourished, overworked stomach and intestinal tract to dispose of as best they can. Small wonder the colon, which used to be called the "garbage can" of the body, is now referred to as the "cesspool."

Milk, so often considered the elite of the protein foods, is loaded with extra salt (milk is naturally high in sodium), preservatives, milk curdling agents, artificial color and artificial flavors. Milk processors are not required to list additives on the package or carton. Random tests through the years have revealed such preservatives as formaldehyde in milk. The process of homogenizing distorts the cream molecule to make it something not found in nature and so not properly digestible. And pasteurization does not kill all the bacteria. Recent tests have revealed that pasteurized milk, probably not handled carefully, has many times over the amount of bacteria of certified raw milk. New-born calves raised on whole, raw milk thrive, while those fed pasteurized milk die about six weeks after birth.

Perhaps you say. "Oh, but children and adults are not calves." To which must be rebutted, nor are infants calves. They are babies who were intended to nurse mother's milk—quite different from cow's—until they are a year old, at which time they no longer need baby food. Not only may milk and milk products cause problems for older children and adults, such as constipation and mucus in the sinuses, bronchia, vagina and intestines, they are the greatest single cause of cataracts. Let me point out that over half of the population tests sensitive to dairy products because their bodies have lost the ability to form the enzymes necessary to digest them. Even those who can may have degenerative problems resulting from a slime-coated, constipated colon from taking mucus-causing milk foods.

I hear countless people wail at the thought of giving up cheese. "But I LOVE cheese. It couldn't be bad for me!" All we can say is, after you've been on the cleansing diet of Phase VII for a time and are feeling great, try a meal of milk or cheese. Just milk or cheese. Then skip the next meal. Or eat the milk or cheese meal at night and skip breakfast. If no problem of any kind occurs after 18 to 30 hours, ole! Milk and natural cheeses are for you. They're either for you or against you. There's no half way between.

In homogenized milk, the fat molecules are changed, broken down into small, foreign particles not found in nature. The body was not made to handle them. They are prone to lodge in the walls of the arteries, causing circulation and heart problems. If you insist on milk in which much of the nutrition is destroyed, take skim milk.

Best of all, drink goat milk. The cream particles are smaller, it's more nutritious for humans than cow milk and much easier to digest and assimilate. Many people who cannot take cow milk can take goat milk and cheese. It's up to you to find out what agrees with you and your family. Remember that we, as adults, must take the responsibility for maintaining or restoring our own good health and that of our children.

If you are absolutely sure that milk agrees with you, that it does not cause gas, mucus, constipation, excess sinus or vaginal discharge, or a hacking bronchial cough, headache or diarrhea flare-ups (the main milk-caused problems), then drink *raw* milk. Make your own cottage cheese and yogurt or buy from a dairy that produces such products without additives.

Experiment with tofu, the soy cheese, after you've ascertained you are not allergic to it. (Many are.) Learn to make seed cheeses, spreads and seed "yogurt" (See *The UNcook Book*). Cultivate a taste for nuts and seeds—they are not as expensive as meats and cheeses, considering pound-for-pound nutrition. There is no moisture waste to nuts and seeds and they need no preparation for eating unless you wish to make something special of them.

You may be wondering about whole grain breads, pies, cakes, pastries, cookies and crackers made at home. They are fine if free of additives, if you can digest them and if you have neither arthritis nor another allergy caused by them. Allergists tell us at least sixty-five percent of the people in the United States are allergic to wheat. At least forty-five percent are allergic to corn. Undetected allergies can be an insidious cause of all sorts of degenerative disease. However, when such grains are sprouted and eaten raw, or made into dehydrated crackers and cookies, they usually do not cause allergies. They digest easily because the starches are converted to fruit sugars and the proteins to amino acids. This makes them all essentially pre-digested. Anyone getting off of hard-to-digest cooked grains, especially wheat, will find a dramatic increase in energy and a feeling of well being.

What we drink may also greatly affect our health. The number one beverage sold today to the unsuspecting or uncaring public is carbonated drinks. The only good they provide is liquid to help flush out all the bad in them . . . a dubious role. The caffeine over-stimulates and is addictive. The sugar and the damaging artificial color and flavor subtly suppress health by displacing good foods like raw fruits and vegetables. (Caffeine also occurs in many bakery products—reportedly to enhance the flavor. What it certainly does is add to the addiction of bakery goodies and cakes.)

What of the non-cola and sugarless drinks? Little if any better. They still have artificial color, artificial flavor and carbonation plus traces of harmful chemicals.

Again we all wail, "But processed foods taste so *good*." Yes, the food industry spends millions of dollars in research and development to make them delicious. In fact, that is goal number one in the industry. Goal two is to make them spoil proof. How well they succeed! Ants and insects won't eat them. Mice, rats and raccoons take one sniff and look further. Sometimes dogs and cats, reared on processed pet foods, will eat some of it. This contributes to digestive or skin or other slow-acting illness for them.

Here are some simple guidelines to quickly and easily help you climb on the Bandwagon to Health:

1. Eat only all natural food—if insects and animals won't eat it, we don't.
2. Drink only pure well, mineral or distilled water.
3. Look forward to your mini-vacation of daily exercise.
4. Think well of others, and make an end to complaining.
5. Give thanks daily for food and shelter, for friend, family and foe and the love and forbearance to enjoy and to cope with them all.
6. Cultivate forgiveness of others and ask God to bless them.

7. Declare goals and an overall plan for your life, but live a day at a time, as though it were your last, in love and praise.

Remember: the day you are in, the "now," is what is vital. Yesterday is a memory, tomorrow a plan. Declare this day, this present, this NOW, the best of your life!

# Dynamic Natural Food Alternatives

*" . . . and the fruit thereof shall be for meat, and the leaf thereof for medicine."*

*Ezekiel 47:12*

How delightful today to be able to provide ourselves with an all-natural feast at all times. Daily we give thanks for the Garden-of-Eden foods that grace our table. There is infinite variety, wholesome earthy tastes and delightful flavors, all with maximum healing and health-giving nourishment. By living on an all-natural diet, our bodies stay clean and free from disease.

We are listing here foods for radiant health. Most are readily available in grocery stores, supermarkets and co-ops, in health food stores, natural grain stores, Oriental food stores, fresh produce markets and farmers' roadside stands. In the Appendix we have listed a few dealers in natural staple foods who sell by mail order. All of these foods offer full natural flavor, joyful eating, high nutrition and oftentimes low cost. We've classified them for easy reference.

## Proteins—Plant

| Grains (Cereal) | Seeds | Nuts | Legumes |
|---|---|---|---|
| Barley | Amaranth | Almond | Alfalfa |
| Millet | Buckwheat | Cashew | Beans (all kinds) |
| Oats | Flaxseed | Brazil | Clover |
| Rice | Pumpkin | Filbert (Hazelnut) | Lentil |
| Rye | Sesame | Macadamian | Garbanzo |
| Triticale | Sunflower | Pecan | Peas (green and |
| Wheat | | Pine (Pinon) | chick) |
| | | Pistachio | Peanuts |
| | | Walnut | |

The most nutritious way to eat these, the most energy-giving, the tastiest and the easiest to digest are as sprouts.

# Proteins—Animal Products

## For a Modified Vegetarian Diet

| | | |
|---|---|---|
| Cow Milk | Yogurt | Natural Cheeses |
| Goat Milk | Kefir | Eggs |

## For a Non-Vegetarian Diet

| | | |
|---|---|---|
| Beef | Chicken | Fish, salt water |
| Lamb | Turkey | Fish, fresh water |
| Rabbit | Other fowl, wild and domestic | |

*Note: Pork, some birds and all shellfish are not recommended because they are scavengers with unclean flesh. Very grave, sometimes fatal illnesses can be caused by eating them.*

# Carbohydrates—Starches

| | | |
|---|---|---|
| Whole Cereal Grains | Carob | Legumes |
| Root Vegetables | Poi | Seeds |
| | Arrowroot | Nuts |

*Note: Sprouts of the seeds and grains give more nutrition and contribute to a cleaner, better digestion.*

# Carbohydrates—Fruits

## Sweet Fruits

| | | | |
|---|---|---|---|
| Banana | Melon (cantaloupe, etc.) | Date | Most other |
| Papaya | Sweet pear | Raisin | dried fruits |
| Zapote | Sweet grape | Fig | Avocado (non |
| Persimmon | | | acid, unsweet) |

## Semi-Sweet Fruits

| | | | |
|---|---|---|---|
| Apple | Grape | Blueberry | Apricot |
| Pear | Pineapple | Peach | |

## Tart or Acid Fruits

| | | |
|---|---|---|
| Blackberry | Loganberry | Cranberry |
| Strawberry | Citrus Fruit | Current |
| Raspberry | Pomegranate | Tomato |

# Dark Green Leafy Vegetables

Leaf Lettuce
Romaine
Iceberg Lettuce
Butter (Bib, Boston) Lettuce
Kale
Celery

Dandelion
Collard
Spinach
Chard
Dill
Bok Choy

Mustard
Beet Top
Cauliflower
Broccoli
Artichoke
Okra

Carrot Top
Turnip Top
Radish Top
Lambs Quarter
Comfrey

# Oils and Fats

**Cold Pressed Oils**
Safflower
Sunflower
Pumpkin Seed
Flaxseed

Peanut
Soy
Olive
Sesame

**Animal fats (soft)**
Butter
Chicken or Goose fat
(from organically grown
birds)

# Seasonings and Condiments
## (Preferably home-produced, fresh or dried)

Parsley
Onion Tops
Celery Seed, Leaves
Dill Seed, Weed
Chinese Parsley
Savory

Peppermint
Spearmint
Vanilla Bean Pod
Oregano
Caraway Seed
Corriander

Dulce
Papaya Seed Pepper
(See Part III)
Sage
Rosemary
Poppy Seed

# Sweeteners

Honey
Maple Sugar,
 Syrup
Molasses
Blackstrap
Barley Malt
 Syrup, Powder

Mexican Piloncillo
 (or S. American Panela)
Treesweet (from Tree Tea)
Cinnamon bark
Raw Cane Juice

Carob (Raw and Toasted
 Powder, Pod Bits)
Sweet Rice Extract
 and syrup

# Herbal Teas
## Non-Sweet

Camomile
Comfrey
Lemon Grass
Shave Grass
Hierba Mate

Spearmint
Peppermint
Red Clover
Alfalfa

Jamaica
Ginseng
Corn Silk
Pau d'Arco

## Naturally Sweet

Cinnamon Bark      Sassafras      Licorice
Tree Tea      Sarsaparilla      Carob

These herbal teas are a few of the better known and tastier ones of literally several hundred kinds made from leaves, barks, flowers, pods or stems from every part of the world. Some of the above-mentioned teas are tasty and pleasant. Some are exotic. They all may be efficacious in maintaining or helping to regain one's health.

Each culture the world over has had its special herb teas for healing illnesses. Modern science now recognizes this. For many years, the United Nations has sponsored scientists to search the earth for medicinal plants from which potions, extracts and teas can be made for healing. Science, not always using the wisdom of the ages, is beginning to accept and prescribe it. God's words of truth and wisdom are coming into their own.

# What About Natural Food Supplements?

(About Noah) "*And take thou unto thee of all food that is eaten and thou shalt gather it to thee; and it shall be for food for thee and for them.*"

*Genesis 6:21*

Although God gave no cause originally for nature's diet to be supplemented, He did provide a few concentrated foods for man's greater strength, health, longevity and enjoyment. Then man began to alter nature in the mid-eighteenth century. By the nineteenth century—as a result of altered, highly concentrated, nutritionless foods as sugar at a cheap price—our nation's health embarked on a gradual, subtle, health-suppressed course. With even cheaper sugar and early addiction to it, plus polished rice and white flour, health began a slallom fall into degenerative disease. Each decade new, unheard-of diseases appeared. Atherosclorosis was diagnosed about 1910 when white flour was first bleached. "Sugar diabetes" was identified in the early twenties.

Today, because of nutrient-depleted soils, herbicides, insecticides and the long periods of time transporting produce from farm to supermarket, foods are far less nutritious than they were at the turn of the century. Add to this a polluted environment that causes our bodies to demand more vitamins, minerals and enzymes for withstanding it. It's no wonder many of us may need food supplements. Fortunately there are a number of complete, natural, concentrated foods (not pills or capsules), that are readily digested, mild-tasting and easy to work into one's daily menus. Here is a discussion of them:

1. **PRIMARY YEAST** (grown on molasses), called *nutritional* yeast to distinguish it from bakers' (bread) yeast. It contains all essential nutrients except vitamin C. It is known for its high content of the B vitamins and the anti-cancer mineral, selenium. Less celebrated although equally important is a full range of other necessary minerals. There are other factors—micronutrients—as yet unidentified in yeast that make it a powerful substance for preventing and recovering from disease. Morning sickness of very

early pregnancy is almost immediately relieved by taking yeast which is high in vitamin B. The nausea of motion sickness and chemotherapy is also relieved by this vitamin. Although yeast is available in capsules and tablets, it is better to take it in powder form. Tablets have to have binders, so often cornstarch plus other excipients that tend to suppress health. Some people are allergic to these excipients. Capsules are made of gelatin plus a hardening factor and may interfere with digestion. A person needing this supplement for recovery rarely will take enough pills or capsules to correct the problem. If a physician or nutrition-oriented therapist recommends a rounded tablespoon of yeast with each meal, the patient would have to take twelve or fifteen tablets or capsules to get that much.

2. **SPIRULINA PLANKTON** is a blue-green, fresh water algae, that grows in a few natural lakes like Lake Texcoco near Mexico City and Lake Chad in Africa. It is also cultivated in man-made tanks in the United States, Korea and Japan. It vies for top place as the most concentrated source of $B_{12}$, with about twice the amount found in liver. It is loaded with B vitamins, including folic acid, so necessary for many functions of the body, and the complete range of essential minerals. Lastly, it is extremely important for its high content of chlorophyl, an effective nutrient for healing all kinds of diseases.

3. **KELP,** the plant that grows abundantly in the sea, is optimally rich in minerals, every known kind with nature's balance. Kelp is prescribed for its content of iodine, iron, calcium, magnesium, potassium and manganese, to mention a few. Easily assimilated because of its organic nature and its balance, it heads the list of source-of-mineral supplements.

4. **BEE POLLEN,** perfect in nutrition, is food for the angels. It contains all the nutrients essential to man. High in the B vitamins, pre-digested and tasty, it needs little or no doctoring with other foods to make it delicious to eat. Bee pollen is as varied in its semi-sweet taste as are the flowers over the various climates of the world. Children develop beautiful, healthy minds and bodies, athletes increase their endurance, housewives find an end to their "fatigue syndrome," men discover new energy, the elderly experience quality-of-living and strength . . . all with a few teaspoonsful a day of wondrous bee pollen.

5. **ROYAL JELLY,** the food for the queen bee, is almost as good as bee pollen. Although not quite as nutritionally balanced as bee

pollen, it nevertheless is a fantastic concentration of the B vitamins. Sold in capsules, it makes a good travel supplement. It can be chewed out of the capsule so the capsule can be spit out. Persons too ill to take food can be massaged with royal jelly mixed with a few drops of oil. According to dermatologists, the skin readily absorbs such nutrients when rubbed at least twenty times.

6. **MOLASSES,** a concentrated sweet, is nevertheless so mineral-rich that even a teaspoonful a day, taken over a period of time, can correct mineral deficiency. The many minerals in raw sugar end up in blackstrap molasses.

7. **DULSE,** dried sea lettuce full of minerals, should be in every kitchen. Twelve times more nutritious than the average garden vegetable, it is an inexpensive food to supplement a diet. Mild and pleasant tasting, it can be added to salads, casseroles, seed-meat patties, tacos or any dish of vegetables. It can be bought whole, (dehydrated) or finely ground for easy dispensing in a large-hole shaker.

# Kitchen Equipment that Works Magic

*"For it is God which worketh in you both to will and to work for His good pleasure."*

*Philippians 2:13*

Recently a feature article writer asked to interview us in our kitchen. After viewing our counters of a few bowls, a tray of jars of sprouting seeds and hand and electric appliances, he asked us what was the most special piece of equipment we used. Without much deliberation we answered that it was our small collection of knives. He looked disappointed until he understood a little more about the preparation of a meal in a mainly raw foods kitchen.

Our knives harvest crops of earth-grown sprouts. They stem, cut, peel, core, chop, scrape, shred and slice. Although we do use such electric appliances as a blender, a grinder that also juices, a juicer and a seed mill, we have to use knives to prepare foods for those machines. And knives, with the use of muscle and a little more time and effort, can do much of what the machines do. Knives should be sharp. We use an emery stone to keep a good edge on them.

Here's a list of cutting knives that daily meet our food preparation needs. There are many more kinds that do special things, but beyond a point, a collection of knives becomes just that, and does not get used.

1. Paring knife, straight edge, three and a half inches long.
2. Paring knife, five inches long, slightly rounded at the top.
3. Paring knife, short, heavy duty, sturdy point for such cleaning and cutting as roots or gouging coconut out of the shell.
4. Medium-sized chopping knife.
5. Long-bladed, fairly heavy duty knife for cutting open melons, winter squash, etc.
6. Long, very sharp serrated knife for slicing breads, harvesting wheat grass, slicing tomatoes and shredding cabbage.

We have more knives but they mostly lie in a drawer. The knives a person uses to prepare foods are as personal as one's lipstick or shave cream. We make our list known simply because we are often asked.

Many gadgets that used to take up precious space in our small kitchen long ago gave way to stainless steel bowls that stack. This resulted in some beautiful empty spots on shelves and in drawers. We learned to prepare all our foods and make all recipes with hand equipment, partly to see if it could be done without sacrificing quality in the end product, partly to give ourselves time and experience to select the right appliance for our use before we spent a great deal of money. Electric appliances are not absolutely necessary, but they are a great time and labor saver. Sometimes we think of them as expensive. Yet the total cost of the four appliances we feel as necessary for us to have, is less than our kitchen range—which we scarcely ever use except to boil water.

Here are some appliances of great help to people following an all-natural diet.

1. Blender, any one of several name brands that serve well for making seed milk (cantaloupe and watermelon), very creamy guacamole, fruit smoothies, green drinks (chopped green vegetables with water, then strained) and so on.

2. Powered grinder with grain grinding attachment (Wheatena-Choprite by Sundance listed in Appendix). This is the only type of appliance that effectively juices wheat grass. (An old-fashioned hand grinder can be used. When the wheat is ground, it can be put in double nylon net or an old nylon stocking and the juice squeezed out.) The grinder is excellent for juicing fruits and vegetables. It presses out the juice, the ideal way to conserve nutrients. If we could have only one appliance, it would be this powered grinder with it flour-making grain grinder attachment.

3. Seed mill for making seed meal and for pulverizing nuts. (See Appendix.) We make lots of seed "cheeses," spreads, salad dressings and nut butters.

4. Heavy duty blender, like Vita Mix, for making frozen fruit ice creams and sherbets, for grinding grains, for juicing and for blending sprouted grains for making Essene breads and raw crackers. All of these things, except grain grinding, can be done in small amounts in an ordinary blender. The heavy duty is a great time saver in its performance and its design for easy cleaning.

5. Champion and Norwalk appliances do a variety of things. Before buying, each person will want to investigate the possibilities and limitations. Neither of these two appliances juice wheat grass effectively, but they make excellent sugarless fruit "ice creams," and do a host of other things.

6. Juice extractor as Acme or Oster. Ours is a centrifugal force design which inevitably destroys some of the vitamins and en-

zymes by oxidation. These types of juicers are fast and otherwise efficient. When short of time, we use ours. Otherwise we use the Wheatena-Choprite.

If you prefer to employ hand methods, you can use a hand grinder, mortar and pestle, a stainless steel, very fine and sharp grater (squeeze grated vegetables through nylon net for juice), chopping board, knife and so on, at very little cost and little chance of trouble with a breakdown or with replacement. You can choose your own way of preparing the recipes in this book. They are that easy.

# Make Your Kitchen Your Garden

*"He who gathers in summer is a son who acts wisely,*
*but he who sleeps in harvest is a son who acts shame-*
*fully."*

Proverbs 10:5

Indoor gardening is our greatest daily thrill. At night we drop seeds into a crystal bed of water and by morning life wells up in tiny buds that promise succulent leaves and stems. We wash them, tipping them to drain and receive the fresh air. Our light-drenched kitchen is filled with the spirit of creation, with renewal, with contentment and with love.

Wherever we go, we "plant" our garden around us. No place is too small, no room too bare to accommodate our precious, budding, growing seeds. Whether you live in Maine, Hawaii or Oklahoma—in a mansion, a house, apartment, condominium, room, cabin or tent—you can grow a garden:

We use the simplest, most inexpensive equipment, mainly because we frequently find ourselves living in everything from the mansion to the tent and from Washington to Mexico. Inexpensive jars, rubber bands, nylon net or old panty hose top the jars. Used cafeteria or oven trays serve as planters for soil-grown sprouts. They carry well, can be acquired almost any place and can be discarded with little loss as we move on.

Here is a comfortable, inexpensive list of equipment you will need to start your indoor garden:

1. Wide mouth glass jars: 1 pint, 1 quart or 1 gallon. (Pint jars for one person, quart jars for two to four persons, gallon jars for from five to ten persons.)
2. Nylon net, plastic screen wire, cheesecloth, nylon panty hose or plastic or metal screen lids.
3. Dish drainer and drip tray or deep pan (we like a square plastic dishpan) with metal, plastic or wood-slat grill for leaning and draining the jars of washed sprouts.
4. Eight or ten cheap cafeteria trays or sheet baking pans. (If you

plan to grow wheat grass every day, you will need eleven or twelve as a minimum for that project alone. We use trays as darkening lids over the sprouting seeds. If you use black plastic covers to keep seeds in the dark, you'll need only seven or eight trays for the growing of the grass.)

5. Two metal—never plastic because earth worms can't live in toxic plastic—garbage cans with holes bored six inches apart, bottom and sides. (Small can for one person, medium can for two to four persons, large can for more.) It is not necessary to have garbage cans for composting your growing (potting) soil, but advisable. They are tidy and convenient. They can sit just outside your back door, on your back porch, on the balcony of your condominium, or in a closet or service corner of your apartment or room. Or you can use a commercial house or apartment composter, or make a compost pit outdoors. They are all good.

6. Hand trowel.

7. Wheelbarrow, wooden mixing box, old bathtub, black plastic sheet, small tarpolin or whatever for mixing soil.

8. Dark-colored kitchen towel. (We like blue, the color of strength, and green, the color of vibrant life.)

9. Serrated knife.

This equipment will supply your needs for a complete kitchen garden. However, if you prefer more sophisticated materials for sprouting, draining and growing, you'll enjoy shopping for them in garden shops and health food stores.

The next step in realizing your kitchen garden is learning where to buy seeds and grains to sprout. Do not expect to buy them in a nursery. They may be sprayed with harmful insecticides. Here is a list:

1. Buckwheat, hulled—co-op (CO), natural grain shop (NGS) or health food store (HFS).

2. Buckwheat, unhulled for growing—CO, HFS and NGS.

3. Corn, special for sprouting—HFS.

4. Corn, popcorn (all popcorn sprouts)—HFS, CO, NGS.

5. Legumes, domestic beans and peas—CO, HFS, NGS.

6. Legumes, imported and special (Mung beans, adzuki beans, cowpeas, garbanzos, dahl and black beans)—CO, HFS, Oriental shops (OS).

7. Sesame seeds—HFS, CO, NGS.

8. Pumpkin and squash seeds—HFS, CO, NGS.

9. Sunflower seeds, hulled—HFS, CO.

10. Sunflower seeds, unhulled—HFS, CO, NGS.

11. Flaxseed—HFS, CO.

12. Vegetable seeds, garden type—cabbage, radish, watercress—HFS.

13. Cereal grains (wheat, rye, barley, hulled oat, rye, rice)—CO, NGS, HFS.
14. Triticale (see Glossary)—CO, HFS, NGS.
15. Millet (see Glossary)—CO, HGS, NGS.
16. Fenugreek (see Glossary)—HFS, CO.
17. Chia (see Glossary)—HFS, CO.
18. Amaranth (see Glossary)—Walnut Acres, Penns Creek, PA 17862.

When you have your equipment and seeds, you are ready. Start your sprout garden with a few of the easy-to-sprout seeds or grains. If you are familiar with alfalfa and mung beans, begin with them. Read the sprouting table on the following pages, measure your seeds, place them in jars, cover the jars with net or screen, wash and drain the seeds two or three times, then submerge them with the purest water available, with the water line an inch or two above the seeds. Set the jars upright in your draining tray and place the tray in a warm, out-of-the-way but not out-of-sight spot. Cover with the dark towel.

You don't want to forget to drain, then wash and drain the seeds again when the time comes. Some people reserve a cupboard for sprouting, or the unused oven. We set ours in an available space by the refrigerator where a bit of warmth from the motor keeps the temperature just right for our cool, northwest climate. Fit your sprouting to your work habits and your kitchen space, or lack of it. If your climate is a warm one, a spot near a window might be better, or even on a porch or room on the shady side of the house.

When you're well into sprouting seeds, you'll want to start to grow plants in soil. If you don't have composted soil or top or potting soil from the nursery to start with, you can prepare your own rich soil. Here's how:

- Decide where to mix a two-and-a-half gallon bucket of dirt—driveway, sidewalk, patio, black plastic spread on the lawn, wheelbarrow, box, or in your kitchen sink or laundry tub (lined with heavy plastic that extends six inches beyond the rim).
- Add to the dirt 1 cup bone meal, ½ gallon steer manure from the nursery and 2 gallons peat moss or fine humus like leaf mold. Mix thoroughly.
- Spread an inch of this rich soil on one of your planting trays and pat down with your hand. The level of the dirt will be a little higher than the edge of the tray. With a pancake turner or your hand, pat the dirt away from the edge of the tray, making a small ditch all around for the extra water, should you sprinkle a little too much. It is ready to be well watered for planting.

With your soil prepared, your next step is to sprout your unhulled buckwheat or sunflower seeds.

For these soil-grown sprouts, you will have to provide a little more space. We dedicated a small metal kitchen bar stool bought at a thrift shop and a wee spot in the bathroom for the covered-tray sprouting period. On the stool, we stack the trays that are covered with an inverted tray. When the growth of the longest sprouting tray of seeds pushes up the lid a fraction of an inch, we remove it and put the tray of pale plants in daylight—a shelf in the service room, or a small table in the dining or living room. These trays of lush plants are beautiful, especially as they turn green in an hour or so. They are decorative, healthful and interesting to watch in their rapid growth. They always create conversation among guests.

Let's say you plan to plant seeds in the evening after work. The day before you plant your first tray of buckwheat (for "lettuce") or sunflower seeds (for "sun sprouts") or wheat, put one cup of seeds and two cups of cool water in a quart jar for soaking overnight (8-12 hours). Next morning drain, wash and drain, leaving the jar up-side-down at a 45° angle for the day in a cool spot. If possible, wash and drain one more time as soon as you return home.

Approximately twenty-four hours after putting the seeds to soak, you are ready to plant. Sprinkle your tray of soil until it is shiny wet. Then spread the seeds evenly over the surface. Sprinkle lightly and cover with an empty tray. Place it in the spot you've designated for sprouting and leave until the top tray is lifted up part of an inch. (About three days). Then it is ready for daylight. Introduce it to full sunlight gradually over a day or two. Water every day with house plant watering can or pitcher, or small jar with holes in the lid. Buckwheat, sunflower seeds and wheat are treated the same.

If every day you plant a tray of sunflower seeds, buckwheat seeds or wheat, always put the newly planted tray on the bottom of your stack of covered, sprouting trays, keeping them in order. The most recently planted, put on the bottom. The next most recently planted on top of it, and so on, with the longest planted one always on top.

Now that you've begun your indoor gardening, you should start composting soil in one of your garbage cans. (You can mix more dirt, bonemeal, steer manure and peat moss, in the proportions given and store all in the other can to use until the can of compost is ready in four to ten weeks, depending on the weather.) In cold climates, composting can be done when the soil is warm enough for the vegetable matter to break down with the rotting process. At all times keep compost quite warm.

When your tray gardens are harvested, dump the used soil in your compost can or outdoor compost pit. Each day add your food garbage—peelings, leftovers, outside leaves, wilted vegetables, eggshells, cooking and/or soaking water (if you don't drink it yourself!)—to the compost. Now and then sprinkle more dirt over it, enough to cover the garbage. Keep tightly lidded. When your can is one-fourth full, add a few earth worms. By now you are a full-fledged, indoor gardener! Enjoy! Rejoice!

A word about harvesting your crops. When these little plants are three to four inches high, they are a gorgeous mass of small, succulent leaves, with only a few black hulls clinging to them. Pick off the hulls. Then with one hand holding a bunch of plants three inches across, cut the stems just above the level of the soil, using your serrated knife. Rinse in cold water. They are ready to eat in or as the most delicious salad ever.

Sunflower seed lettuce or sprouts are grown and harvested in exactly the same way as buckwheat. However, the plants are different. Buckwheat, a smaller seed, yields a smaller stem and leaf. Sunflower, even the smaller, black hull variety more readily available in the eastern part of the United States, is twice or three times the size of buckwheat. Here in the west we find mainly the large striped, sunflower seed yielding thick, juicy stems and leaves.

Wheat grass is highly nutritious, a complete food and very healing. Wheat grass juice helped one of us get over cancer and both of us surmount many health problems. We grow a tray yielding eight to ten ounces of juice every day for the two of us. During summer we grow a tray every other day because we eat more green vegetables and need only two to three ounces a day. We use red winter wheat for growing, white spring wheat for Essene bread.

Wheat grass stubble can grow into a second crop which will yield 4 to 5 oz. of juice. When we are too busy to plant, we water the stubble of a cutover tray and add a little liquid organic plant fertilizer.

We cannot over-stress the indoor growing of sprouts, whether in jars and/or soil. Sprouts are the elite of foods. Well chewed, they cause no digestion problem. They are readily absorbed by the body. The starches (hard to digest) are converted to fruit sugars which are pre-digested. The proteins convert to amino acids, also pre-digested. Since the body expends little energy for digestion, it has abundant energy for activity. This is why after eating sprouts and fruits, you never have that sluggish, sleepy-headed feeling that drags one down with a case of the "Blahs."

The word *pulse* of the Bible, the food Daniel ate for a keen mind, a high spirit and glowing health, really means sprouts. Pulse means life flow. Daniel ate a diet of life flow, according to God's instructions.

# Sprouting Chart

| Seeds | Sprouting Equipment | Soaking Time | Water, Rinse and Drain | Sprouting Time |
|---|---|---|---|---|
| Adzuki | Jar | 8 hours | 3 times/day | 3-4 days |
| Alfalfa | Jar | 8 hours | 3 times/day | 4-5 days |
| Almond | Paper Towels | 4 hours; drain | Sprinkle 3 times/day | 3-5 days |
| Barley | Jar | 8 hours | 3 times/day | 3-5 days |
| Beans | Jar | 8 hours | 3 times/day | 3-5 days |
| Buckwheat | Jar or Paper Towels | 8 hours | 3 times/day | 2-3 days |
| Cabbage | Jar | 8 hours | 3 times/day | 3-5 days |
| Chia | Flat bottom bowl | | Sprinkle 3 times/day | 4-5 days |
| Clover | Jar | 8 hours | 3 times/day | 1-2 days |
| Corn | Jar | 8 hours | 3 times/day | 4-8 days |
| Fenugreek | Jar | 8 hours | 3 times/day | 3-4 days |
| Flax | Jar or Paper Towels | 4 hours | 4 times/day | 4-5 days |
| Garbanzo | Jar | 8 hours | 4 times/day | 2-3 days |
| Garden Cress | Jar | 8 hours | 3 times/day | 3-4 days |
| Lentil | Jar | 8 hours | 3 times/day | 3-4 days |
| Millet | Jar | 8 hours | 3 times/day | 3-4 days |
| Mung Bean | Jar | 8 hours | 3 times/day | 3-5 days |
| Mustard | Paper Towels | 4 hours; drain | Sprinkle 3 times/day | 3-5 days |
| Oat | Jar | 8 hours | 4 times/day | 2-3 days |
| Pea | Jar | 8 hours | 3 times/day | 3-4 days |
| Pumpkin | Jar | 8 hours | 3 times/day | 3-4 days |
| Radish | Jar | 8 hours | 3 times/day | 2-4 days |
| Rice | Jar | 8 hours | 3 times/day | 3-4 days |
| Rye | Jar | 8 hours | 3 times/day | 2-4 days |
| Sesame | Jar | 8 hours | 3 times/day | 3-4 days |
| Soybean | Jar | 8 hours | 4-5 times/day | 2-4 days |
| Sunflower | Jar | 8 hours | 2 times/day | 24-36 hrs. |
| Triticale | Jar | 8 hours | 3 times/day | 1-3 days |
| Wheat | Jar | 8 hours | 3 times/day | 3-5 days |

1. Alfalfa, clover and rye sprouts, when an inch or two long, may be greened in daylight or sunlight for two to four hours for salad greens.

2. Beans include white, black, haricot, kidney, fava, pinto, navy, lima and broad.

| Harvest Length | Yield | Suggested Use |
|---|---|---|
| 1″ | ½ c. seeds, 2 c. sprouts | Salads, sandwiches, juices |
| 1½″ to 2″ | 3 T. seeds, 1 qt. sprouts | Salads, juices, soups, sandwiches |
| ⅛″ to ¼″ | ½ c. seeds, ¾ cups | Snacks, use in almond recipes |
| | | |
| ¼″ | 1 c. seeds, 1 c. sprouts | Breads, soups, cereals |
| ½″ to 1½″ | 1 c. seeds, 4 c. sprouts | Vegetable loaves, salads |
| ⅛″ to ½″ | 1 c. seeds, 3 c. sprouts | Salads, cereals, cookies, breads |
| ½″ to 1″ | ¼ c. seeds, 1¼ c. sprouts | Salads, seasonings, sandwiches |
| ½″/ 2 leaves | 2 T. seeds, 3 c. sprouts | Soups, dips, spreads |
| Seed length | ½ c. seeds, 1¼ c. sprouts | Salads, spreads, soups |
| ½″ | ½ c. seeds, 1 c. sprouts | Soups, salads, cereals |
| ½″ | ¼ c. seeds, 1 c. sprouts | Salads, vegetable loaves |
| 1″ to 2″ | 2 T. seeds, 1½-2 c. sprouts | Curries, spreads, salads |
| ¼″ to ½″ | ½ c. seeds, 1 c. sprouts | Soups, marinates, salads |
| 1½ in. greened | 1 T. seeds, 1½ c. sprouts | Slaw salads, seasoning |
| 1″ | ½ c. seeds, 1 c. sprouts | Salads, soups |
| ¼″ | 1 c. seeds, 3 c. sprouts | Breads, cereals |
| 2″ to 2½″ | 1 c. seeds, 4-5 c. sprouts | Salads, vegetable dishes |
| 1″ to 2″ | 1 T. seeds, ¼ c. sprouts | Salads, seasonings |
| | | |
| ¼″ to ½″ | 1 c. seeds, 2 c. sprouts | Breads, cereals, cookies |
| Seed length | ½ c. seeds, 1 c. sprouts | Soups, vegetable dishes |
| ¼″ | 1 c. seeds, 2 c. sprouts | Snacks, salads, candy |
| ½″ to 1″ | 1 T. seeds, ¾ c. sprouts | Seasonings, salads |
| Seed length | 1 c. seeds, 2½ c. sprouts | Vegetable loaves, cereals |
| Seed length | 1 c. seeds, 2-3 c. sprouts | Breads, granola |
| Seed length | 1 c. seeds, 1½ c. sprouts | Cheese, cookies |
| 1″ | 1 c. seeds, 2-3 c. sprouts | Tofu, cheese, salads |
| ⅛″ to ¼″ | 1 c. seeds, 2 c. sprouts | Vegetable "meat", salads |
| Seed length | 1 c. seeds, 2-3 c. sprouts | Breads, cereals |
| Seed length | 1 c. seeds, 3-4 c. sprouts | |

3. Cabbage and other members of the same botanical family - broccoli, brussel sprouts, cauliflower, collards, and kale.

4. Garbanzos are also called chickpeas and gram.

# Multi-Miracles of Dehydrated Foods

*"And let them gather all food of those good years that come and lay up corn . . . and let them keep food in the cities."*

Genesis 41:35

Of the various ways to preserve foods for storage, dehydration and drying are the best. They conserve the most nutrition. The process of freezing destroys a little more than dehydration. Canning destroys the most nutrition of all. Dehydration has other advantages. It costs less, keeps without refrigeration, stores in the least space and requires a minimum of labor.

Vitamins, except for C, are not lost in dehydration. Nor are most enzymes. In the process of drying, the fruit sugar is increased. This makes dried foods a little higher in calories of the best, most energy-giving, digestible kind.

Most of us think of dried foods as supplies for pack-trips and hiking, or for snack foods. And they are wonderful for such purposes. But wonderful they are, too, for delicious basic and exotic recipes in the kitchen, for sweeteners, for treats, for travel and for holiday fare.

### There are several ways of drying foods

● Sun-drying is the oldest, perhaps the best—certainly the cheapest—way to preserve foods. Fruits or vegetables should be washed, carefully dried on an old turkish towel or absorbent cloth, sliced thin and laid in a single layer on drying trays or boards. (Do not use iron unless rust free and very slightly oiled, or aluminum.) Cover with nylon net or very thin gauze or cheese-cloth and set in the sun after morning dew is evaporated. Bring in the house before the cool of evening. Sun drying, depending on the intensity of the sun and the climate, will take from one to three or four days to be completely dry. The day you store your dried food, place it in the sun fifteen or twenty minutes to dry out any re-absorbed moisture it might have gotten in a moist kitchen or early morning exposure. Store in tight lidded glass jars, pre-washed plastic bags or containers that can be sealed, or tins with tight lids.

*Note: New plastic is toxic. When it is washed and dried two or three times it ceases to be an allergen for most people. It will have lost most of its toxic gas.*

• Dehydration with a commercial or hand-made dehydrator offers many pluses. It is convenient, it saves time and work, it controls the heat used in the process. We find that dehydrators with a fan work very efficiently because they circulate evenly the warm air. Some report they use less electricity. A thermostat or some form of temperature control on a dehydrator is advisable since temperatures above 104° start to destroy enzymes. We like to dehydrate at 90°, letting the dehydrator run day and night until the foods are dry. There are many different kinds of dehydrators on the market, from small, round counter top models to larger square and oblong ones with many trays. Each person will want to shop for the size, price and kind that best suits his or her needs. Some do-it-yourself people make very good dehydrators. Plans for such creations can be obtained from the *Mother Earth* News Magazine and *Sunset Magazine.*

• Oven drying requires only a little more time and doing than drying with a dehydrator, but is not difficult. Place the two or three racks in the center slots of your oven. While preparing your food, set the oven at 200° and turn on. When the oven has reached that temperature, turn off the heat and put your fruits, vegetables, sprouts or leaves in and prop the oven door open slightly. I use a piece of crumpled foil. Leave until the oven cools to near room temperature. Take out the trays of drying foods, re-set the oven and put the food in again when the heat goes off. Repeat this act all through the day and until you retire. Propped open, the oven light will keep the temperature at a low-dehydrating level. Next day repeat the oven-drying process until the food is thoroughly dry, then store. Sometimes one can supplement oven-drying with sunshine.

Once you get into dehydrating and drying foods, you will find all sorts of ways to increase your nutrition and decrease your spending. For instance, dried carrot tops make an interesting seasoning and a tasty, beneficial tea. Extra leaves of all kinds get dried at our house, as comfrey, raspberry and violet leaves for tea. In the dehydrator they dry in a few hours. Or hanging in the woodshed (leaves should not be sun-dried) they yield quantities of dried leaves for tea blends and for hostess, birthday and Christmas gifts. We raise so much parsley, dill, camomile and mint in pots as ornamental shrubs and food that we often have to dry the extra crop to save it. And how wonderful to have those things safely stored and ready to use at little or no cost!

Books have been written on dehydration (See Bibliography). However, most people, once started, like to think up their own ways of managing a dehydrating program. Here are a few more suggestions:

1. Onion tops, finely chopped, celery leaves, dill weed and/or seed, tender radish tops, the early, tender, seeding head of any garden vegetable. Mix or keep separate to use as seasoning for salad, casserole, stew, nutmeat loaf, tacos, etc.
2. Fruit leathers made by pureeing, dehydrating, chopping fine and using to flavor such mild teas as mint, comfrey, camomile, lemon grass, shave grass and rose hips (from your garden). With a touch of spice you have a creation!
3. Extra summer garden vegetables dehydrated for winter soups and stews.

Learn the easy art of dehydrating. You'll be excited, inspired and satisfied. You save money. You won't work hard. And you *will* have fun!

# Stable Emotions and a Positive Attitude

*"And we know that all things work together for good to them that love God . . ."*

*Romans 8:28*

New energy! Clarity of thinking! A sense of being at peace! These things are released to you as you finish the Phases and Chapters. What is more wonderful than reaching the goal of being a truly Complete Person nutritionally, spiritually and physically?

Our body is the temple of the Living God. Cleansed from the chemical impurities most people ingest, it no longer causes us to be hypersensitive; nor do we have caffeine jitters. Exercises help us to become more relaxed, trim and vigorous. And that leads to a big boost in our self-confidence. Knowing our body is in good condition and attractive to behold is a natural high for most of us.

With a new well-tuned machine in optimal running condition, how can we expect anything but the best? In Proverbs 17:22 we are told, "A merry heart doeth good like a machine . . ." And why shouldn't we be merry? The condition of our thoughts has a direct relationship to actual conditions in our lives! That's why it is so important to practice "positive expectancy." When we look for the best, we find it in everything and everyone. As we claim it, we are one with God and the depth of our trust and faith leads us down roads we never even knew existed.

The human mind is a miraculous mechanism. It gives us whatever we dwell on. This is a universal law. If we hold high thoughts and anticipate our lives being surrounded with positive results, that's what we get! So if we constantly feed our minds good, loving thoughts, we find the quality of our life will be in proportion to those thoughts. Try it. It works when we let go of negativism. It frees our resentments and releases bitterness. Then we can more fully let our own special light shine. We can approach each day with thanksgiving and joyful anticipation.

Another law of nature is temperance in all things. Exercise that is vigorous but not excessive is the ideal. We can strive for a natural, balanced diet, sparingly eaten. (Gluttony is considered by many physicians to be the greatest single cause of illness.) Hard work and play are vital . . . but need to be stopped before the onset of fatigue.

By observing these truths, we have a strong body—joy abundant—contentment—strength—and a clear mind to walk the way to fulfillment of the radiant life God intended for us.

# Transitional
## Recipes for
### A New You

*"And God said, Let the earth bring forth grass, the herb yielding seed, and the fruit tree yielding fruit after his kind, whose seed is in itself, upon the earth: and it was so."*

*Genesis 1:11*

The foods in Part III are made up of both cooked and uncooked recipes. As you will see, there are more uncooked ones than cooked. In the first place, cooked recipes already far outnumber the uncooked. Secondly, uncooked foods are thirty to ninety percent more nutritious. And thirdly, there are many more different taste thrills and adventures in delicious eating with original, raw, gourmet food recipes. They open up a whole new world of eating with resultant good health and the fulfilling experience of expansion of mind and spirit.

# WHOLE GRAIN BREADS AND CRACKERS

Natural whole grain breads are made with whole grain flours and only a few basic ingredients. They help to keep a menu simple, natural, digestible yet delicious.

The breads are coarser than soft commercial ones. They are firm, chewy and nutty tasting, the flavor getting even better the more you chew—in contrast to white flour products that lose their flavor after chewing a few times.

Use only one grain for a recipe. Do not mix grains. Each grain is a special taste treat. This helps you to follow a food rotation plan.

Do not use coated baking pans or pan spray to keep breads from sticking. Both are toxic, expecially when heated.

## BASIC WHOLE GRAIN BREAD (BAKED)

6 C. whole grain flour (rye, barley, wheat or triticale)

2 T. dry bread yeast

¼ C. oil

¾ t. salt or ½ t. salt and 1½ t. S.A.

½ C. warm water

3 to 3½ C. room temperature water

Dissolve yeast in warm water and set aside. Mix S.A. and salt with flour. Add oil, moistened yeast, ⅔ of the water and stir, adding more water to make a heavy but stirable dough. Place in warm spot and allow to rise once or twice (1 to 2 hours), stirring down each time. Pour into two 4½" x 8" pans, oiled and floured, and let rise an hour. Bake at 325° for 45 minutes or until bread starts to pull away from pans. A toothpick stuck in should come out with a tiny bit of crumbs on it. Turn on a side until nearly cool. Remove from pans and serve, or finish cooling, wrap in wax paper and store.

*Note: Use this same recipe for Barley Bread. Rye Bread. Wheat Bread and Triticale Bread.*

# BASIC WHOLE GRAIN CRACKERS (BAKED)
## (One Recipe Makes All)

2 C. whole grain flour

1½ t. S.A. and ½ t. salt

1 T. bread yeast, dry

1¾ C. lukewarm water

2 T. oil or butter

Dissolve yeast in lukewarm water. Set aside. Mix flour, salt and S.A. Add yeast mixture into flour and stir until very smooth. Dough should be about like thin pancake batter. If not, add a bit more water. Drop by teaspoon onto well oiled cookie pan. Or pour batter in thin layer over the pan. Bake at 350° for 20 to 25 minutes. Cut the layer of crackers immediately on removing from oven. Take all crackers off pan with pancake turner. Cool on racks. Store while cool and crisp in tight containers.

*Note: Everyone likes these nutritious, delicious crackers. We bake for company and family. Rarely are any left to store!*

*Note: These crackers can be made with any cracker seasoning: 1 t. dill weed or seed, or 1 t. celery powder, or ½ t. onion powder, or ¼ t. garlic powder, or ⅛ t. cayenne, or 1 t. caraway seed.*

# BASIC SPROUTED GRAIN CRACKERS (RAW)

For super nutrition, taste, energy and health, we make these dehydrated crackers. One recipe makes all kinds: rye, buckwheat, oats, barley, wheat, triticale, corn. You can make them plain or add seasonings as in the baked crackers. The consistency of the dough may be a little different because of the individuality of the grains. And the amount of water may have to be adjusted slightly, depending on the length of the sprout. (The longer the sprout, the more water is contained in the grain and the less water is needed in the recipe.) The basic recipe for these raw crackers calls for the sprout on the grain to be about the length of the grain. If it's longer, it's still all right but the flavor will be slightly stronger.

148

# RAW SPROUTED GRAIN CRACKERS
## (Dehydrated)

4 C. sprouted grain (2 C. before sprouting)

1 C. water or grain soak water

1½ t. S. A. and ½ t. salt

Seasonings to taste

Blend sprouted grain with water, salt and seasonings for 15 seconds for a coarse textured cracker or 25 seconds for a fine textured cracker. Spread on cellophane or plastic wrap-lined dehydrating trays or cookie pans. Or drop by teaspoon in circles. Dehydrate at 100° or less. When almost dry, lift plastic and crackers off the tray, turn over and peel the plastic off the crackers. Cut in squares if in sheets, and finish dehydrating. Store in tight containers in a cool place.

## AMARANTH STOVE-TOP MUFFINS

2 C. amaranth flour

½ t. salt

3 T. oil

3 eggs

½ C. warm water

1 T. dry bread yeast

1 C. water

Dissolve yeast in warm water and set aside. Mix amaranth flour and salt, then add oil, eggs, water and yeast mix. Stir well. Set aside for 1 to 2 hours in warm spot or overnight at room temperature. 15 or 20 minutes before baking, stir down and let rise. Bake in 2½ to 3 inch cakes in 400° skillet for an unusually tasty, chewy, nutty, pancakelike stove-top muffin.

# SEED AND NUT MEAT LOAVES, PATTIES, AND PIZZA

# NUT MEAT LOAF OR PATTIES

½ C. sprouted garbanzos

1 large carrot

1 C. nuts

2 T. flaxseed meal

½ to 1 t. celery, caraway,
poppy or dill seed

½ t. salt

1 to 2 T. water

Onion if desired

Grind or put through food processor the garbanzos, carrot and nuts. Add the flaxseed meal, sprinkled, seasoning seeds, salt and water and onion, if used. Mix as you would any meat loaf. Form into a loaf, allow to season 30 minutes, chill and serve. Loaf can be warmed over hot water if desired.

# SEED MEAT LOAF OR PATTIES

½ C. sesame seed meal, or
buds

1 comfrey root, size of small
carrot

2 stalks celery

1 C. alfalfa sprouts

1 T. chopped onion
(optional)

Meat seasoning to taste

½ t. salt

Grind, put through food processor or chop finely, comfrey root and celery. Mix thoroughly with other ingredients, form into loaf or patties, set aside to season. Chill or warm and serve with or without seed or tomato sauce.

*Note: Seed and nut meat loaves, patties and croquettes can be made in infinite variety of the many vegetable, seed and nut combinations. The ingredients that make them stick together nicely, besides flaxseed and comfrey root, are slippery elm powder, chia and psyllium seed and agar-agar, 1 t. to ¼ C. hot water, dissolved.*

# PIZZA CRUST (COOKED)

1½ C. whole grain flour

¼ C. oil

3 to 4 T. water

½ t. salt

Mix flour and oil, add salt and water. Work into a dough. Put into a pizza pan and bake until light brown. Serve with cooked pizza filling.

## PIZZA CRUST (RAW)

1½ C. sprouted, dehydrated buckwheat flour

¼ C. oil

½ t. salt

Mix flour and salt, then add oil, mixing thoroughly. Firmly pat into pizza pan. Make raw pizza filling (see Seed and Nut Meat Loaves), pour over the crust and let stand 30 minutes. Warm over hot water and serve for a surprising treat.

## VEGETARIAN PIZZA FILLING

1½ C. ripe tomatoes

1 T. each of chopped bell pepper, celery, onion

4 T. flaxseed meal

⅛ t. cayenne

¼ t. oregano

¼ t. thyme

½ t. salt

1 C. tofu

2 T. tamari sauce

½ C. pecans

Blend all together, except tofu, pour into raw pizza crust and chill for eating raw, or warm over hot water for eating. Just before serving, scatter 1 C. of tofu ½-inch cubes marinated in tamari sauce, and pecans, over the top.

# SOUPS, COOKED AND RAW

## BEET SOUP

1 C. finely grated beets

2 avocados

1 celery stick, chopped

1 t. S. A. and ¼ t. salt

1½ C. water

Scoop avocado out of shells into blender. Add celery, salt and water and blend. Set over hot water if warm soup is desired. Or chill and serve, with the grated beets sprinkled over top. Very attractive and delicious.

# TOMATO SOUP

2 C. tomatoes, mashed

2 T. pecan butter

1 C. alfalfa sprouts

Salt to taste

Blend tomatoes, with skins, pecan butter and salt. Serve hot or cold with chopped alfalfa sprouts spread over top.

# CELERY SOUP

2 C. chopped celery

2 C. seed, nut or coconut milk

1 T. tamari sauce

1 T. butter

½ t. onion powder (optional)

Blend, heat in double boiler to 110° and serve in heated soup cups.

# FRESH GUMBO SOUP

1 large carrot, diced finely

2 C. water

1 stalk celery, chopped

1 C. okra, thin-sliced

1 to 2 T. butter

Boil carrot in water 5 minutes. Cool to 140°. (You can't quite hold your hand on bottom of pan.) Add celery, okra and butter. Heat a little more if cooled below 100° and serve in preheated cups.

# SALAD DRESSINGS

## GUACAMOLE DRESSING

1 small to medium avocado

½ t. salt

½ t. dill weed

1 dash onion powder (optional)

1 T. lemon juice or apple cider vinegar

Mash and/or puree until smooth. Toss salad with the dressing or serve the dressing on top.

# SESAME SEED DRESSING

1 C. sesame seed meal

Water or oil to make creamy

½ t. celery seed

¼ t. oregano

1 pinch of cayenne (optional)

Mix water or oil in the sesame meal, adding only enough to make a heavy cream, then stir in the seasoning. Serve over or tossed in the salad. Refrigerate if made in advance.

# SUNFLOWER SEED DRESSING

Make the same as sesame seed dressing using different seasonings as papaya seed pepper, thyme and garlic.

# ALMOND BUTTER DRESSING

1 C. almond meal (or any nut meal)

Water or oil to make a cream

Pinch of salt (optional)

Mix the water or oil in the meal, a bit at a time, to make a thick cream or thin cream, as is desired. Serve over fruit or vegetable salads.

# FLAXSEED DRESSING

½ C. flaxseed meal

2 T. oil

⅓ C. water

½ t. dill weed

½ t. rosemary

½ t. chopped chives or onion

Pinch of cayenne

Mix the oil and water with the meal and add the other ingredients. Set aside 10 or 15 minutes to thicken. If a thinner dressing is desired, add more water. Serve or refrigerate for later.

## OIL AND VINEGAR DRESSING

½ C. apple cider vinegar

½ C. olive oil

½ t. celery salt

½ t. marjoram

½ t. onion powder (optional)

¼ t. fresh ground pepper

¼ t. dry mustard

½ t. caraway seed

1 T. sesame seed, meal or whole

Put all ingredients in a bottle with tight lid, shake well and pour over or toss with a vegetable salad.

## TOMATO PURÉE DRESSING

2 ripe, medium tomatoes

2 T. flaxseed or 1 T. psyllium seed meal

½ t. celery powder

½ t. dill weed

½ t. dry mustard

¼ t. salt or 1 t. S.A.

Pinch of onion and/or garlic powder

Peel and mash tomatoes. Add the flaxseed meal and seasonings. Mix thoroughly or blend. Chill and serve or refrigerate. Will keep up to 24 hours.

# CREATIVE SALAD COMBINATIONS

The charming thing about salads is that no two need be exactly alike. Here are some exciting combinations. (Most everything raw, of course.)

No. 1 Zucchini
     Okra
     Jícama

With tomato dressing

No. 2 Carrot
     Eggplant
     Alfalfa sprouts

With oil and lemon dressing

| No. 3 Shredded cabbage<br>Shredded yam<br>Raisins | Almond butter dressing |
|---|---|
| No. 4 Spinach<br>Bean sprouts<br>Tomato | Sesame seed dressing |
| No. 5 Okra<br>Jícama<br>Avocado | Olive oil and vinegar dressing |
| No. 6 Shredded beets<br>Chopped celery<br>Tomato | Avocado (guacamole) dressing |
| No. 7 Fenugreek sprouts<br>Bean sprouts<br>Zucchini | Sunflower seed dressing |

# SALAD SPROUTS

| | |
|---|---|
| Bean (Adzuki) | Lentils |
| Bean (Mung) | Cabbage |
| Alfalfa | Radish |
| Clover | Buckwheat |
| Chia | Garbanzos |

*Note: Chia, a fantastic energy food, is best sprouted in a flat bottom dish or pie plate. We use a large corning dish. Spread the seeds thickly (single layer) over the bottom and sprinkle with enough water to wet them. Keep moist by frequent sprinkling through the day. Roots form first, pushing up the mucilaginous seeds in little humps. Next come the tiny green leaves, two on a stem. When they are about ½ inch high, they are ready to eat, roots, black seed hulls and all.*

*Garbanzos, after overnight soaking, can be washed and drained several times for a day or, because they spoil rather quickly, put in the refrigerator to continue to sprout very slowly. Use them for several days, a few tossed in a salad, a casserole, soup or other vegetables.*

# CEREALS

## GRANOLA

1 C. popcorn, buttered or plain

1 C. Buckwheat Crunchies

⅛ t. salt

½ C. raw sunflower seeds or ¾ C. budded, dehydrated sunflower seeds

1 C. oatmeal

1 T. honey or molasses

1 T. oil or melted butter

Mix dry ingredients in large bowl. Warm oil or butter mixed with honey or molasses over pan of hot water. Dribble over dry mix, stirring constantly. Serve or store in cool dry place for no more than a few days. Better to refrigerate in tight container.

## SPROUT CEREAL

1 C. sprouted buckwheat

¼ C. sprouted (barely budded) sesame

½ C. budded sunflower seeds

¾ C. wheat bran or fresh wheat germ

½ C. boiling or cool water

Pour boiling water over bran and set aside 10 minutes. Or pour cool water over wheat germ and set aside a few minutes. Then mix in the buckwheat, sesame and sunflower seeds. Serve with fresh fruit or dried fruit, as is or reconstituted.

*Note: This is excellent camp cereal. Sprout before going or during camp in plastic bags.*

# GRANOLA BARS AND COOKIES

Granola bars, each kind a balanced meal of all essential nutrients of high quality, can be made of any sprouted, dehydrated grain flour. Some kind of seed mill or fine grinder is necessary to make the flour of dehydrated grains. The advantages of sprouted seed flours are numerous: (1) They contain many times the amount of vitamins of plain traditional flours. (2) They are ready to eat raw. (3) They keep well, stored in tight containers in a cool dry place. (4) They taste so good, a nut-like flavor quite different from ordinary flours.

It is well to sprout, dehydrate and store all kinds of grains—wheat, rye, barley, oats, buckwheat, triticale, corn, millet, rice—ahead to have ready to grind into flour and make into granola bars, cookies, pie crusts, pizza crusts and even breads, all on short notice. We have grains sprouting most of the time to keep our crash food preparation program functioning at all times. That way we are always ready for drop-in guests and spur-of-the-moment potlucks, picnics, etc.

Granola bars are surprisingly high in proteins, minerals, enzymes and vitamins, particularly B vitamins, and comfortably low in carbohydrates.

A rye granola bar 1½" x 3" x ½" has approximately 100 calories.

## GRANOLA BARS

2 C. sprouted, dehydrated grain flour (rye, wheat, oats, barley or buckwheat)

1 t. S.A. and ¼ t. salt

1 C. sticky dates, ground

¾ C. nuts or sunflower seeds, ground

2 T. molasses or honey

1 T. liquid lecithin

1 T. cold pressed oil

¾ t. vanilla

¼ t. almond extract

Mix flour, S.A. and salt. In large bowl mix molasses or honey, lecithin, oil, vanilla and almond extract, then add nuts and dates, mixing thoroughly. Add the flour mixture, bit at a time, working with heavy spoon or by hand. Press into 9" x 9" pan, cut into bars and serve or store in tight container in the refrigerator.

*Note: If dough is too stiff for you to manage, sprinkle a few drops of water over it and work in. Instead of bars you can make "sausage" rolls and slice, or make 1½" balls and flatten. Children love to make them.*

## MORE GRANOLA BARS (COOKIES)

Take any combination of the following basic ingredients for other variations:

| Dried Fruits | Nuts | Seeds | Sweeteners | Grains |
|---|---|---|---|---|
| Dates | Walnuts | Sesame | Honey | Rye |
| Figs | Filberts | Sunflower | Molasses | Oats |
| Raisins | Pecans | Pumpkin | Barley Malt | Barley |
| | Almonds | | Rice Syrup | Wheat |
| | | | | Buckwheat |

*Note: Coconut can be used in granola bars instead of nuts if there is no chance that water will be added. When raw coconut gets and stays moist for more than thirty minutes to an hour, it tastes like soap. Though mildly so, it alters the excellent taste of the bars.*

# WHOLE GRAIN CAKES

The cakes in this section can be made with either sprouted grain (rye, wheat, triticale, barley) which has more B vitamin in it, or regular whole grain flour. However, you will need to remember that regular flour is a little heavier, which means a slight alteration in the balance of flour and water. In the recipes that follow, sprouted grain flours have been used. If you use regular whole grain flour—and they taste just as good—use ¾ cup to 1 cup of sprouted grain flour. For example, the 2 C. of sprouted grain flour in the recipes would be changed to 1½ C. of regular whole grain flour.

Like whole grain breads, whole grain cakes are firmer and chewier than conventional ones. They are oh-so-satisfying and good!

In the recipe for the 2 C. of whole grain to be sprouted, you will need to substitute 2 C. whole grain flour and 1½ C. water for the ¾ C. water of the sprouted grain recipe.

## CAROB CAKE (BAKED)

2 C. (scant) grain (before sprouting)

¾ C. water

1 C. carob

¼ t. salt

3 t. baking powder

3 T. honey

2 eggs

4 T. oil

1 t. vanilla

½ t. almond extract

Blend sprouted grain and water at high speed until very smooth. Or twice grind and add water. Add oil, vanilla, almond extract and honey. Mix carob, salt and baking powder then stir into grain mixture. Separate yolks from whites of eggs and beat into batter. Whip whites to stiff froth. Fold in batter. Pour into 9" x 9" oiled and floured pan. Bake at 350° for approximately 40 minutes. Cool upside down on rack before taking out of pan.

## Carob Chip Topping

¾ C. water

1 or 2 T. butter

1 t. vanilla

Pinch salt

1 T. honey

1 T. cornstarch or arrowroot

3 T. cool water

½ C. carob chips

Bring water to boil. Dissolve thickening in water and add slowly to boiling water, stirring constantly. When thickened remove from heat, cool slightly and add butter, vanilla, salt and honey, stirring. When cooled add ½ C. carob chips. Stir and spread on top of carob cake. Serve or chill and serve. (Nuts may be added if desired.)

# BIRTHDAY FRUIT CAKE (BAKED)

(Made with rye, wheat or barley flour. Our favorite is rye.)

1½ C. flour

3 t. baking powder

1 t. S.A. and ¼ t. salt

3 T. oil

3 T. honey

2 eggs

½ C. chopped, dehydrated apricots

½ C. dehydrated sweet cherries or raisins

½ C. chopped dates

½ to 1 C. chopped nuts

½ t. mace or cinnamon

⅓ C. water

Mix flour, baking powder, salt and spices. Make a cup-size hole in the flour. Add the rest of the ingredients in order given. Stir well. Bake in 5" x 9" loaf pan at 350° for 40 minutes. Cool partially on a side, then turn out for finishing. We serve this cake with thick cream when all the family comes home. All ages love it. With fresh fruit in season or fruit juice, it makes a completely balanced meal and so-o-o-o delicious.

# ORANGE CAKE

3 C. whole wheat flour

5 t. baking powder

¼ t. salt

1½ C. orange juice

¾ C. oil

¾ C. honey

4 eggs

1 t. vanilla

*Rosita Rangel*
*San Carlos*
*Guaymas, Sonora, Mexico*

Mix the flour, baking powder and salt in a large bowl. Separately mix together the orange juice, oil, honey, eggs and vanilla, then add to the flour mixture. Stir in well then beat for a minute or two. Pour into two deep layer pans or 3 shallower pans that have been oiled and floured slightly. Bake in a moderate oven 45 minutes for a surprisingly different, fine-textured and delicious cake.

# CARROT CAKE

2 C. whole wheat (or other whole grain) flour. (We like barley.)

4 t. baking powder

⅓ t. salt

Spice to taste (nutmeg, mace)

2 eggs

½ C. honey or molasses

4 t. oil or butter, melted

½ to 1 C. nuts or sunflower or pumpkin seeds

½ C. fine chopped dates, figs or raisins

2 C. grated or ground carrots

½ t. vanilla

1 C. water

Mix dry ingredients. In a hole made in the center, drop all the other ingredients in order given. Bake in 8" x 11½" pyrex pan at 350° for 40 minutes or until inserted toothpick comes out clean. Cool in the pan. Serve plain, with the carob chip sauce, or with or without the carob chips (coconut is an interesting substitute) or with whipped cream. Again, this can be a complete meal except for vitamin C. Serve fresh fruit or juice with the cake for that vitamin.

# BREAKFAST CAKE

(Made with rye, barley, wheat or triticale)

2 T. bread yeast

½ C. lukewarm water

1½ C. whole grain flour

1½ t. S.A. and ¼ t. salt

1 C. chopped dates, figs or apricots

½ C. raisins

3 T. oil

2 T. honey if dates or figs are used, 3 T. if apricots are used

¾ C. chopped walnuts

2 eggs

½ t. vanilla

½ t. almond extract

½ t. nutmeg

¼ t. allspice

1¼ C. water

Dissolve yeast in lukewarm water and set aside. In large bowl, mix flour and salt/S.A. Make a cup size hole in flour, add dried fruits and mix. Then add the rest of the ingredients, stirring until batter is smooth. It will be fairly stiff. Oil and flour-dust a 9" x 9" pan and pour batter in. Let rise 20 to 30 minutes. Bake at 350° for 35 minutes. Serve hot or cool, with or without whipped or plain, thick cream. Served with fresh fruit in season or fresh fruit juice, it makes a memorable breakfast, completely balanced.

# ICE CREAMS

The so-called ice creams that follow have no cream at all, although cream can be added or used as an alternative to avocado. (½ C. cream instead of 1 medium avocado.) These recipes are made in a heavy duty blender such as Vita Mix or, half at a time, in a regular kitchen blender.

We made fruit ice creams, all different kinds, using bananas as a base until we discovered that one of us was terribly allergic to bananas. (They caused depression, irritability and energy loss.) Since we and our family look forward to our twice-weekly treat of ice cream with great anticipation, we have to come up with an alternative to bananas. The first three recipes that follow are made with that alternative. The next two are made with bananas for the majority that can eat them. And the last two, hopefully for everyone, are surprisingly different and fantastically good also.

# BLACKBERRY ICE CREAM

2 C. frozen blackberries,
heaped up

½ C. water

¼ C. honey

1 medium apple, chilled

1 medium avocado, chilled

Dissolve honey in water. Core and dice apple into blender. Scoop avocado out of shell into blender. Add honey-water, then frozen berries and blend at high speed until a thick cream. Serve in dishes chilled in deep freeze. (This recipe can be followed for making any kind of berry ice cream.)

*Note: For making this ice cream in a regular type blender, put half the berries in a flat bottom stew pan, pour half the honey and water over it along with half the avocado and apple and let sit a minute or two. Then mash with potato masher and blend. You might have to add a little water. The ice cream will be soft. Serve in freezer-chilled dishes. Instead of serving with cake or cookies, try sprinkling with Buckwheat Crunchies or budded sunflower seeds for a complete meal. (Make other half of the ice cream.)*

# PEACH ICE CREAM

3 C. frozen peaches

½ C. water

3 T. honey

1 medium avocado

Mix water and honey. Scoop avocado out of half shells into the heavy duty blender, add honey-water, then peaches. Blend at high speed and serve in chilled dishes.

*Note: Almost any frozen fruit can be used in this recipe instead of peaches. Only the honey needs to be increased or decreased, depending on the sweetness of the fruit. For instance, persimmon ice cream takes only a T. Plums and cherries take 4 T. honey*

# TART APPLE ICE CREAM

3 medium frozen apples

½ small can frozen apple juice, partially thawed

1 medium avocado

2 to 4 T. water

Scoop avocado out of half shells into heavy duty blender. Add icy juice and blend, using extra water if needed. Serve at once in freezer-cold dishes. If using regular kitchen blender, follow Blackberry Ice Cream recipe instructions.

162

# BLUEBERRY ICE CREAM NO. 1

3 frozen bananas

2 C. blueberries or 2 C. frozen blueberries and 3 ripe bananas

1 T. honey

3 T. water

Dissolve honey in water. Cut bananas (frozen or fresh) into heavy duty blender, add blueberries (fresh or frozen) then the honey-water and blend. If too much for blender, add water, tablespoon at a time, testing the blender each time to see if there is enough water. Serve in chilled dishes. (If regular blender is used, proceed according to instuctions under recipe for Blackberry Ice Cream.)

*Note: Banana can be used as the base for any fruit ice cream.*

# BLUEBERRY ICE CREAM NO. 2
(Made in Champion or Norwalk)

4 frozen bananas

1 C. blueberries

Cut each banana in 4 pieces. Feed into the hopper, alternating with fresh or frozen blueberries. Catch the ice cream in chilled bowl or individual dishes. Serve at once.

# UNIQUE BERRY ICE CREAM

3 C. frozen, unsweetened strawberries

3 T. flaxseed meal or 2 T. psyllium seed meal

2 T. honey

½ C. plus 2 T. water

Tiny pinch salt

2 t. safflower oil

Dissolve honey in water then stir in flaxseed or psyllium seed and salt. Set aside 5 or 10 minutes to allow mixture to thicken. Put all ingredients in heavy duty blender and blend to a stiff cream, adding extra water if needed. (If making in regular kitchen blender, follow Blackberry Ice Cream recipe instructions.)

# UNIQUE ORANGE-APRICOT ICE CREAM

2 C. (packed) ripe apricots or reconstituted dried apricots, frozen

3 T. flaxseed meal or 2 T. psyllium seed meal

1 T. honey

½ C. plus 2 T. orange juice

Tiny pinch salt (optional, but it adds to flavor)

2 t. safflower oil

Dissolve honey in orange juice then stir in flaxseed or psyllium meal and salt. Set aside 5 or 10 minutes to allow mixture to thicken. Put all ingredients in heavy duty blender and blend to stiff cream, adding extra water if needed. Serve at once. (For making in regular blender, turn to instructions given in Blackberry Ice Cream recipe.)

# HEAVENLY FRUIT PIES AND CRUSTS

Summer is a good time to treat your family and friends to fresh fruit pies, the epitome of elegance among desserts. They are *so* delicious and nutritious, and untouched by heat. They can be made with reconstituted (24-hour soaked) dried fruits or fresh ones—plums, peaches, apricots, prunes, apples, persimmons, bananas. With only a slight change because of different juice content, one recipe fits all. There can be variations in the crust, too. Our favorites are sprouted, dehydrated rye, oats, barley and buckwheat, for extra nutrition and taste. An equally tasty crust is made from oat flour (found at health food stores) or made from rolled oats ground into flour in your blender or by crumbling it with your hands. When using very juicy fruits, like most berries, you may need to increase the amount of thickening agent (flaxseed or psyllium meal or agar-agar) by a teaspoonful or so, or pour off a little juice when you crush the fruit for the purée. The very tart fruits like raspberries may need an extra tablespoon of honey, while bananas and persimmons will need one less than the basic recipe. Frozen fruits can be used if they contain no sugar. They should be thawed before using.

Before making the fruit filling for Heavenly Pies, you will need to make the crust. Here is the basic crust recipe that can be changed by selecting a different flour. (Sprouted rye, wheat, oats, barley, buckwheat or oat flour.)

# BASIC PIE CRUST

⅔ C. dehydrated sprouted grain flour

⅔ C. fresh wheat germ or wheat bran

Pinch salt

3 T. melted butter or safflower oil

Mix sprouted grain flour, wheat germ or bran and salt, then add the butter or oil and mix thoroughly. Line a pyrex pie plate with mixture patting down well.

# HEAVENLY RAW APRICOT PIE

10 large or 15 small, very ripe apricots or 1½ C. reconstituted dried ones, drained

4 T. honey (3 T. if dried apricots used)

3 T. flaxseed meal

Pinch salt

1 t. lemon juice

2 T. agar-agar

½ C. hot water or juice drained off apricots, heated

2 ripe but firm apricots

½ C. whipping cream

¼ t. vanilla

1 T. honey

Blend quartered apricots, honey, flaxseed meal, salt and lemon juice a few seconds, or mash with a fork and whip until creamy. Dissolve agar in water or juice, add and mix. Pour into crust and chill for several hours. Whip the cream, stir in vanilla and honey and spread over pie. Slice the apricots and arrange in floral design with a wisp of parsley in the center. This pie draws exclamations from all.

# HEAVENLY FRESH APPLE PIE

First, prepare the crust and *chill*, then make the pie filling.

3 C. chopped or thinly sliced summer apples

2 T. agar-agar

¼ C. hot water

1 C. frozen apple juice concentrate (less if apples are very sweet)

2 T. flaxseed meal

Pinch each of allspice and nutmeg or cinnamon

Dissolve agar-agar in hot water, add to thawed apple juice and pour over apples. Mix in flaxseed meal and spice seasoning. Pour over the crust evenly, and chill. Top with whipped cream. You'll have to repeat this recipe often. It's that good!

# TEA BLENDS FOR FUN

Nothing is more fun than to sit down to an exciting cup of herbal tea with beloved friends or family. It's fun to create blends and try out your ingenuity, or tailor-make something for your own taste. Here are a few ideas to get you started. We find floral teas blend well, grasses blend, and dried fruits go with bark teas which often taste slightly sweet.

## HERBAL TEA BLENDS
1. Sassafras and dried apple bits
2. Sarsaparilla, orange peel and allspice
3. Peppermint, comfrey and/or shave grass
4. Rosehips and dried apricot bits
5. Camomile and elder flower

# GREEN DRINKS

Leaves are for our healing. Perhaps the easiest way to get sufficient chlorophyl and minerals chelated by nature is to make a green drink of them. The nutrients in green leafy vegetables require a lot of chewing to break down the cellulose covering of the cells, and chewing is much neglected by most of us. A juicer or blender helps to break down this barrier to assimilation by the body. Here are a few suggestions to get you started. We always try, regardless of the season, to have some green leaves to include in the drink along with whatever "filler" vegetables we have on hand, as zucchini or winter squash, carrots and other root vegetables.

## GREEN DRINK NO. 1

¼ small head cabbage

2 large carrots

1 bunch spinach

Put through a juicer (Acme, Oster, Champion, Mix Master juice attachment, Wheatena Choprite, Norwalk, etc.) or chop all the vegetables and put in the blender, half cover with water, blend on high speed and strain out pulp.

## GREEN DRINK NO. 2

4 stalks celery with leaves

2 tops of small beets

½ head romaine

Make according to instructions in Green Drink No. 1.

## GREEN DRINK NO. 3

1 medium zucchini

Several large leaves kale

2 bunches dandelion, with root

1 medium carrot

Make according to instructions in Green Drink No. 1.

# RECIPE NOTES IN A NUTSHELL

● Sodium ascorbate (S.A.) is used to salt foods, to help preserve them and to provide vitamin C.

● Apple cider vinegar, preferably aged in wooden barrels (Heinz), is full of nutrients. White synthetic is not. It is good for cleaning windows.

● Sprouted seeds and grains are many times more nutritious than dry ones. They are among the cheapest, tastiest, best foods available.

● Dried fruits, according to recent findings, *do* have more fruit sugar than they did in their fresh state.

● Cold pressed oils, without preservatives and solvents, are not processed with the extreme heat of long shelf life oils bought in supermarkets. They are found in co-ops and health food stores. They still contain the essential oil, lineoleic acid.

- Mock refried beans are first sprouted, then cooked and mashed with a little oil or melted butter. They are delicious!
- Paprika is an excellent, mild condiment very high in vitamin A. We forget to use it often enough.
- Kelp is full of minerals, salt being a predominant one. Many put kelp in their salt shakers as a salt substitute. We did not include it in recipes simply because most people have to learn to like it. However, we recommend it.
- A salt blend that we use and call C-salt is made of equal parts of sodium ascorbate, sea salt, kelp and powdered celery. It is a good partial salt substitute.
- Whey powder, or dehydrated whey, the by-product of cheese (the liquid left when the curd coagulates and is removed), is valuable to those who tolerate milk products. It is a good source of lactobacillus, a culture encouraging beneficial flora of the intestines necessary for absorption of foods. It is high in salt and some other minerals, notably calcium, and contains some protein.
- Sesame seed budding should be stopped (washed, drained, then refrigerated) as soon as the bud appears. The longer the budding sprout grows, the more bitter it will be. Refrigerate and use soon.
- Oatmeal, or rolled oats, by some name brand companies, is subjected to intense heat to give it long shelf life. Buy at health food stores, natural food shops and co-ops where they stock oatmeal that has not been heated too much and so needs to be refrigerated for keeping.
- If the end of a potato grows above ground, it turns green in light and develops a toxic element in it. Cut off this green, poisonous end. Potatoes should not be exposed to light after they are harvested. Store in a dark place.
- When traveling, soak seeds for sprouting (at night) in a plastic bag. Cover seeds in the bag with twice the amount of water, hang up with a safety pin, leaving bag partially open. In morning drain and wash. With pin, poke holes in bag and hang for draining. Wash 2 or 3 times during the day.

*Note: Royal Rule for Recipes—If bugs and animals eat it, then you eat it. If they don't, then avoid it like poison, because it is!*

# Appendix

## VITAMIN AND MINERAL DATA

The vitamins and minerals, their functions, deficiency symptoms and natural sources listed below, are included for reference. It is not our role to advocate supplementing one's diet with them. There is such a great overlap in the causes of deficiencies that only a nutritionally, biochemically-oriented physician or therapist should be consulted to diagnose the problems and prescribe the diet and/or supplements.

Our purpose in compiling the following data is purely educational and informative. We wish, in so doing, to make clear to you, our readers, that foods as they occur in nature —fresh, unfired and unprocessed—contain all nutrients essential for a healthy body. With this in mind, one can use the lists as a guide in planning a diet regimen to fit his or her individual needs.

## VITAMIN A

**Functions:** Essential to membrane tissue and resistance to infections in sinuses, lungs, air passages, gastro-intestinal tract, vagina and eyes; prevents night blindness, sensitivity to light; promotes growth, vitality, appetite and digestion; helps prevent aging and senility; helps counteract damaging effects of air pollution.
**Signs of Deficiency:** Cystitis, sinusitis, bronchitis, gastritis; loss of appetite, retarded growth, eye problems—night blindness, red eyes, bad vision; defective teeth; dry, scaly skin, psoriasis, acne, wrinkles, pimples.

**Sources:** Dark green leafy vegetables, orange and yellow fruits and vegetables such as carrots, yams, cantaloupes, apricots; whole grains, especially wheat, rice and oats, seeds and nuts; sprouts.

# VITAMIN B COMPLEX

In all cooked foods, this brain and nerve-nourishing vitamin complex is partially or completely destroyed, depending on the intensity of heat and time of cooking.

**Functions:** Promotes digestion, growth and appetite; maintains health of nerves and brain; necessary for the quality and quantity of milk during lactation; increases pancreatic secretions, one of which is insulin; maintains adrenal, thyroid, anterior pituitary glands; improves heart and circulation; aids in production of hydrochloric adic; aids in protein-carbohydrate-fat metabolism; helps prevent tooth decay, edema, epileptic seizures, and a host of other degenerative diseases such as arthritis and Parkinson's diseases.

**Signs of Deficiency:** Eye problems (i.e. cataracts); ulcers, loss of appetite, poor digestion, skin eruptions, mental depression, edema, anemia, halitosis, colitis, premature aging and senility, sore mouth and eyes; loss of vigor and weight, constipation, subnormal temperature, pathological disorders of adrenals, thymus, ovaries, spleen, heart, testes, liver, thyroid, kidneys, brain and pituitary; tendency to diabetes, disorders of thyroid, nerves and blood.

**Sources:** Whole cereal grains, especially sprouted, and sprouted seeds and legumes, served raw, dark green leafy vegetables, raw fruits, brewer's yeast.

# VITAMIN C
## (Ascorbic Acid and the Bioflavonoids - C complex)

**Functions:** Essential for good collagen, the "glue" that holds the cells together; necessary for vital functions of all organs and glands, especially adrenals, thymus and thyroid; protects against all stress (physical and mental), toxic chemicals in food, air and water, drugs and such poisons as rattlesnake bite and bee sting; acts as natural antibiotic and general protector against toxic metals, as cadmium, lead, mercury; essential for oxygen metabolism and for healthy teeth and gums; promotes leuocytic and phagocytic activity.

**Signs of Deficiency:** Soft, bleeding gums, decaying teeth, spontaneous bruising and purpura, lowered resistance to all infections and the toxicity of drugs and airborne poisons; skin hemorrhages, nose bleed, anemia, toxic thyroid, premature aging, physical weakness, rapid breathing and heart beat; reduced adrenal secretions; tendency to ulcers, stomach and duodenal. Absence of Vitamin C causes scurvy.

**Sources:** All raw fruits and vegetables, especially red bell peppers, tomatoes, rose hips, citrus fruits, acerola cherries, green leafy vegetables and sprouts.

# VITAMIN D

**Functions:** Essential for the utilization of calcium and other metals by the digestive tract; necessary for proper function of thyroid and parathyroid glands; assures proper formation of bones and teeth in children.

**Signs of Deficiency:** Rickets, tooth decay, pyorrhea, osteomalacia, osteoporosis, retarded growth, muscular weakness, low energy, lack of mineral assimilation and premature aging.

**Sources:** Exposure of uncovered skin to the sun whose rays change the ergosterol in the skin into Vitamin D; fish liver oils, raw milk, egg yolk, sprouted seeds, wheat grass juice, mushrooms.

# VITAMIN E

**Functions:** Provides oxygen to tissues and cells; improves circulation; prevents and reduces scar tissue from burns, surgery and sores; retards aging; lessens menopausal disorders; essential for the health of reproductive organs; serves as an anti-coagulant; prevents death from blood clot; aids circulation; shields lungs and other respiratory organs from air pollution; necessary for treatment and prevention of arthritis, heart disease, burns, asthma, phlebitis, emphysema, varicose veins, leg ulcers, bed sores and a host of other problems; prevents calcium deposits on blood vessel walls; loss of motility of eye lens; aids in lessening arterial hypertension.

**Signs of Deficiency:** Degeneration of coronary system, heart disease, strokes, pulmonary embolism, sterility, pains in muscles, nerve system; eye and cerebral hemorrhage; dermatitis, eczema; fragility of red blood cells.

**Sources:** All raw and sprouted seeds and cereal grains, legumes, seeds, especially flax and nuts; wheat germ if it is no more than 3 or 4 days old (older, rancid germ contains no Vitamin E); eggs, dark green leafy vegetables.

## VITAMIN F

**Fuctions:** Helps to prevent heart disease by lowering blood cholesterol; necessary for function of adrenal and other glands; promotes growth, healthy skin and mucous membranes. Helps in making calcium and phosphorus available to cells, and in protecting from radiation.

**Signs of Deficiency:** Skin problems as eczema, dry skin, acne, fatigue, retarded growth, prostate and menstrual disorders; falling hair, gallstones, constipation, friability of bones (especially in the elderly).

**Sources:** Unrefined, unprocessed vegetable oils such as flaxseed oil, sunflower oil, soy oil, safflower oil and corn oil. Avocado is also a good source of oil.

## VITAMIN G

**Functions:** Growth and development factor; essential to proper calcium utilization and formation of erythrocytes.

**Signs of Deficiency:** Calcium deposits as cataracts of the eye; underdevelopment, anemia, pellagra.

**Sources:** Brewer's yeast, eggs, cereal germ.

## VITAMIN K

**Functions:** Vital for blood clotting and liver function. Called the anti-hemorrhaging vitamin, it also aids in vitality and longevity.

**Signs of Deficiency:** Hemorrhaging anywhere in the body; premature aging and low energy.

**Sources:** Seeds, sprouts, raw milk, egg yolks, alfalfa, kelp. Friendly bacteria in healthy intestines will synthesize Vitamin K.

## VITAMIN T

**Functions:** Helps in correction of nutritional anemia and hemophilia and in forming blood platelets; helps improve failing memory.

**Sources:** Sesame seeds, raw and sprouted; sesame seed butter, some seed oils and raw egg yolk.

# MINERALS

## CALCIUM (Ca)

**Functions:** Vital for all muscle and activity of the body; needed for building and maintenance of bones, for normal growth, heart action, blood clotting; essential for normal pregnancy and lactation, for phosphorus, Vitamins A, C and D utilization; must be present for magnesium to be utilized. There needs to be a balance between calcium and magnesium for both to be used normally by the body.
**Signs of Deficiency:** Fragile, porous bones, heart problems; insomnia, tooth decay, nervousness and irritability, poor growth, muscle spasms, cramps, and rickets.
**Sources:** Sesame seeds (more than in milk), egg yolk, milk and milk products, dark green leafy vegetables such as dandelion, Romaine, spinach, kale, broccoli and brussel sprouts; kelp and sea plants.

## CHLORINE (Cl)

**Functions:** Aids liver in detoxifying the body; necessary for the production of hydrochloric acid which is used in the stomach for digestion of proteins.
**Signs of Deficiency:** Disturbance of levels of fluids in the body; indigestion and poor assimilation of foods.
**Sources:** Kelp, dulse and other sea plants, dark green leafy vegetables, avocado, oats, asparagus, tomatoes, sea fish.

## CHROMIUM (Cr)

**Functions:** Necessary for utilization of sugars; involved with activity of hormones and enzymes; aids in metabolism of cholesterol; identified as glucose tolerance factor; helps regulate serum cholesterol.

**Signs of Deficiency:** Diabetes, hypoglycemia (low blood sugar) and/or hyperglycemia (high blood sugar), heart disease, hardening of the arteries, high serum cholesterol.

**Sources:** Whole cereal grains (preferably sprouted), brewer's yeast, raw sugar cane, mushrooms and liver.

## COBALT (Co)

**Functions:** Combines in hemoglobin-type molecule to synthesize Vitamin $B_{12}$; essential for formation of hemoglobin.

**Signs of Deficiency:** Pernicious anemia.

**Sources:** Comfrey, alfalfa, liver, some green leafy vegetables.

## COPPER (Cu)

**Functions:** Essential for the absorption of iron; helps in development of nerves, bones, connective tissues and brain; aids protein metabolism, maintaining hair color; essential for RNA production.

**Signs of Deficiency:** Anemia, heart and digestive problems, graying of hair, respiration difficulty, hair loss.

**Sources:** Found in such iron-rich foods as legumes (peas, beans, etc.) leafy green vegetables, whole grains and their sprouts, almonds, raisins, prunes, liver.

## FLUORINE (F)

**Functions:** Useful against infections; necessary in formation of healthy bones and teeth; too much, as in fluoridated water, is toxic and causes brown spots on teeth.

**Signs of Deficiency:** Weakened tooth enamel and calcium deficient bones.

**Sources:** Whole grain oats, seeds, carrots, green vegetables, almonds, milk, vegetable tops (especially beets).

## IODINE (I)

**Functions:** Essential for the health and function of the thyroid gland which regulates much of the body's activity, both mental and physical; regulates energy, body weight and metabolism; helps maintain healthy skin.

**Signs of Deficiency:** Enlargement of thyroid gland and goiter; fatigue, loss of sexual interest, anemia, overweight, altered pulse rate, low blood pressure, heart disease and high cholesterol.

**Sources:** Dulse, kelp and other sea plants; green leafy vegetables and green tops of root vegetables (i.e. turnips and beets), pineapple, citrus fruits, watercress, sea foods, fish liver oils and egg yolks.

## IRON (Fe)

**Functions:** Necessary for formation of red blood cells (hemoglobin) which transport oxygen to each and every body cell. Good quality hemoglobin provides resistance to disease and stress.

**Signs of Deficiency:** Anemia, weakness, headaches, pale skin, shortness of breath, difficulty in concentating, lack of interest and vigor, apathy towards sex.

**Sources:** Brewer's yeast, blackstrap molasses, raisins, prunes, nuts, seeds, whole grains, sea plants, sprouts, liver, egg yolks, alfalfa, green leafy vegetables and legumes.

## LITHIUM (Li)

**Functions:** Involved with the involuntary nervous system; aids in metabolism of sodium and its transferance to muscles and nerves.

**Signs of Deficiency:** Mental and nerve problems, especially paranoia and/or schizophrenia.

**Sources:** Sea water, kelp; some mineral waters.

## MAGNESIUM (Mg)

**Functions:** Essential for enzyme activity; aids in body's use of the B vitamins and Vitamin E, fats and other minerals, especially calcium; helps provide good bones and muscle tone; contributes to a healthy heart; balances acid-alkaline condition of the body; helps prevent build-up of cholesterol; necessary for normal, healthy heart function.

**Signs of Deficiency:** Muscle cramps, kidney stones and damage, heart attacks, atherosclerosis, disorientation and nervousness, epilepsia and faulty protein utilization. A prolonged deficiency causes the body to lose calcium and potassium, creating a deficiency in those and other metals; involved in protein synthesis.

**Sources:** Sesame, sunflower, pumpkin seeds, nuts (especially almonds), whole grains, green leafy vegetables (i.e. kale, celery, dandelion, chard and endive), alfalfa, soybean (particularly sprouted), apples, peaches and lemons.

## MANGANESE (Mn)

**Functions:** Vital to enzymes involved with the utilization of proteins, carbohydrates and fats; aids in reproduction; involved with nourishment and coordination responses between brain, muscles and nerves; with the help of choline, aids in digestion and absorption of fats.

**Signs of Deficiency:** Digestive problems, asthma, poor balance, sterility, bone deformity and abnormal growth.

**Sources:** All dark green leafy vegetables, apricots, oranges, blueberries, the outer coat of grains (bran) and nuts, legumes, raw egg yolk, kelp and sea plants.

## MOLYBDENUM (Mo)

**Functions:** Helps prevent copper poisoning (cases of copper poisoning have greatly increased since copper tubing for bathrooms and kitchens began replacing conventional iron pipes); works together with some enzymes in the oxidation process; necessary for carbohydrate metabolism.

**Signs of Deficiency:** "Where molybdenum is lacking in the soil, the land is barren," says Dr. Carl C. Pfeiffer in *Mental and Elemental Nutrients*. Deficiencies have not as yet been positively identified. However, all tissues need a trace of molybdenum. From what is known to date, it seems entirely possible that sexual impotency, dental caries and cancer of the esophagus may be signs of molybdenum deficiency.

**Sources:** (In order of percentage found in foods.)
Whole buckwheat, lima beans, fresh wheat germ, soybeans, barley, lentils, oats, sunflower seeds, whole grain rye and eggs.

## PHOSPHORUS (P)

**Functions:** Works in conjunction with calcium, in correct balance, for formation and maintenance of teeth and bones; essential for normal mental and nerve activities; major involvement with acid-alkaline balance of tissues and blood, and also carbohydrate metabolism.

**Signs of Deficiency:** Weakness, reduced sexual desire, retarded growth, poor bone mineralization, lowered brain and nerve performance.

**Sources:** Nuts, seeds, whole grains, legumes, sprouts, dairy products, dried fruits, egg yolks, and fish.

# POTASSIUM (K)

**Functions:** Prevents overacidity by acting as agent to keep acid-alkaline balance in tissues and blood; necessary for muscle contraction; since the heart is a muscle, potassium is essential to proper heart function, especially the heart beat; necessary for normal nervous system; stimulates endocrine and other hormone production; aids kidneys to detoxify blood. There must be a proper balance between potassium and sodium (salt) for both to function normally.

**Signs of Deficiency:** Edema, sodium poisoning, high blood pressure and heart disease and/or failure; low blood sugar (hypoglycemia), weakness, exhaustion, mental and nervous problems and constipation.

**Sources:** Vegetables (particularly dark green leafy ones), nuts, seeds (sunflower and pumpkin), oranges, bananas and potatoes with peelings.

# SELENIUM (Se)

**Functions:** Has role similar to Vitamin E as anti-oxidant; helps conserve the body's use of that vitamin; protects hemoglobin in red blood cells from oxidation damage; protects against mercury poisoning; helps to prohibit cancer cell proliferation; slows the aging process.

**Signs of Deficiency:** Premature aging, liver malfunction, muscle atrophy.

**Sources:** Brewer's yeast, kelp, sea plants, whole cereal grains, organically grown vegetables and fruits and sprouts.

# SILICON (Si)

**Functions:** Necessary for strong bones, teeth and nails and good hair growth; aids in protecting and healing body against skin problems and irritations in membranes.

**Signs of Deficiency:** Thinning hair, wrinkles, brittle fingernails, osteoporosis, insomnia.

**Sources:** Sprouts (especially alfalfa), kelp, young green plants, strawberries, grapes, beets, almonds, sunflower seeds, steelcut oats (fresh).

## SODIUM (Na)

**Functions:** Sodium, potassium and chlorine maintain osmatic pressure necessary for the absorption of nutrients from intestines into the blood; they maintain body fluids at normal levels; they change into electrically charged ions which transport nerve impulses; sodium must be present for hydrochloric acid production in the stomach; necessary for other glandular secretions.

**Signs of Deficiency:** Although sodium deficiencies are infrequent, they can result from prolonged ingestion of diuretics, excessive perspiration or chronic diarrhea which may cause weakness, heat prostration, nausea, apathy, breathing problems.

**Sources:** Sea water, kelp, sea salt, celery, sea plants, Romaine lettuce, asparagus.

## SULFUR (S)

**Functions:** Essential for beautiful hair, nails and skin, hence called the "beauty mineral". Helps in conserving oxygen in the cells.

**Signs of Deficiency:** Eczema, blemishes, rashes of the skin; brittle nails and hair, problems in joints.

**Sources:** Watercress, horseradish, radish, celery, onion, turnip, nasturtium, fish, soybeans.

## ZINC (Zn)

**Functions:** Vital for synthesis of DNA and RNA and body protein; along with insulin, aids in carbohydrate and energy metabolism; helps the healing of wounds and burns; aids in ridding the body of carbon dioxide; vital in normal growth and tissue respiration, and especially reproductive organs.

**Signs of Deficiency:** Underdeveloped sexual organs, enlargement of prostate gland, birth defects, retarded growth, subnormal sex activity, low resistance to infections, sterility, slow healing of skin diseases, cuts and burns, hair loss, apathy, dandruff.

**Sources:** Sprouted and fermented seeds and grains as in the seed cheeses and Essene breads. Zinc in seeds and grains, "locked" in by phytin, is "unlocked" in sprouting and/or fermenting. Also found in natural seeds (especially pumpkin), brewer's yeast, raw milk, eggs, oysters (highest known source), green leafy vegetables, herring and nuts.

# TABLE OF FOOD COMPOSITION

| FRUITS | Measure | Weight g | Calories | Protein g | Fats g | Carbohydrates g | Calcium mg | Iron mg | Magnesium mg |
|---|---|---|---|---|---|---|---|---|---|
| Apples, raw, whole | 1 med | 130 | 76 | 0.3 | 0.8 | 17.0 | 9.0 | 0.39 | 10.4 |
| Apricots, raw | 1 med | 38 | 19 | 0.4 | 0.1 | 4.1 | 6.5 | 0.19 | 4.6 |
| Avocado | 1 lg | 216 | 361 | 4.5 | 33.0 | 12.0 | 22.0 | 1.30 | 97.0 |
| Banana, raw | 1 med | 150 | 128 | 1.6 | 0.3 | 30.0 | 12.0 | 1.10 | 49.5 |
| Blackberries, raw | 1 cup | 144 | 84 | 1.7 | 1.3 | 17.0 | 46.0 | 1.30 | 45.0 |
| Blueberries, raw | 1 cup | 140 | 87 | 1.0 | 0.7 | 19.0 | 21.0 | 1.40 | 8.4 |
| Cantaloupe, raw | ¼ | 100 | 30 | 0.7 | 0.1 | 7.5 | 14.0 | 0.40 | 16.0 |
| Cherries, sour, raw | 1 cup | 200 | 116 | 2.4 | 0.6 | 28.6 | 44.0 | 0.80 | 28.0 |
| Cherries, sweet, raw | 1 cup | 200 | 140 | 2.6 | 0.6 | 32.0 | 44.0 | 0.80 | 22.5 |
| Cranberries, raw | 1 cup | 100 | 460 | 0.4 | 0.7 | 10.8 | 14.0 | 0.50 | - |
| Dates, dried | 1 med | 10 | 27 | 0.2 | t | 6.3 | 5.9 | 0.30 | 5.8 |
| Elderberries, raw | 1 cup | 457 | 329 | 11.9 | 2.3 | 75.0 | 174.0 | 7.30 | - |
| Figs, dried | 1 lg | 21 | 58 | 0.9 | 0.3 | 13.0 | 26.0 | 0.63 | 14.9 |
| Figs, raw | 1 med | 38 | 30 | 0.5 | 0.1 | 6.8 | 13.0 | 0.23 | 7.6 |
| Gooseberries | 1 cup | 150 | 59 | 1.2 | 0.3 | 14.6 | 27.0 | 0.75 | 13.5 |
| Grapefruit, raw, red flesh, 5″ diam. | 1 med | 260 | 108 | 1.3 | 0.3 | 25.0 | 46.0 | 1.14 | 31.2 |
| Grapes, American Concord | 1 cup | 153 | 106 | 2.0 | 1.5 | 21.0 | 24.0 | 0.61 | 19.9 |
| Grapes, European, Muscat, or Tokay | 1 cup | 160 | 107 | 1.0 | 0.5 | 25.0 | 19.0 | 0.64 | 9.6 |
| Grapes, green, seedless | 1 cup | 200 | 102 | 1.0 | 0.2 | 27.2 | 16.0 | 0.60 | - |

| Phosphorus mg | Potassium mg | Sodium mg | Vitamin A IU | (Thiamine) B$_1$ mg | (Riboflavin) B$_2$ mg | Vitamin B$_6$ mg | Vitamin B$_{12}$ mcg | Folic Acid mg | Niacin mg | Vitamin C mg | Vitamin E mg |
|---|---|---|---|---|---|---|---|---|---|---|---|
| 13.0 | 143 | 1.0 | 117 | 0.040 | 0.03 | 0.039 | 0 | 0.003 | 0.13 | 5.20 | 0.40 |
| 8.7 | 107 | 0.4 | 1,026 | 0.010 | 0.02 | 0.023 | 0 | 0.001 | 0.23 | 0.38 | - |
| 91.0 | 1,305 | 8.6 | 626 | 0.240 | 0.43 | 0.907 | 0 | 0.060 | 3.46 | 31.00 | - |
| 39.0 | 555 | 1.5 | 285 | 0.080 | 0.09 | 0.765 | 0 | 0.010 | 1.05 | 15.00 | 0.33 |
| 27.0 | 245 | 1.4 | 288 | 0.040 | 0.06 | 0.075 | 0 | 0.021 | 0.60 | 30.00 | - |
| 18.0 | 113 | 1.0 | 140 | 0.040 | 0.08 | 0.094 | 0 | 0.011 | 0.70 | 20.00 | - |
| 16.0 | 251 | 12.0 | 3,400 | 0.040 | 0.03 | 0.086 | 0 | 0.007 | 0.60 | 33.00 | 0.14 |
| 38.0 | 218 | 4.0 | 2,000 | 0.100 | 0.12 | 0.170 | - | 0.012 | 0.80 | 20.00 | - |
| 38.0 | 382 | 4.0 | 220 | 0.100 | 0.12 | 0.064 | 0 | 0.012 | 0.80 | 20.00 | - |
| 10.0 | 2 | 82.0 | 40 | 0.030 | 0.02 | 0.040 | - | - | 0.10 | 11.00 | - |
| 6.3 | 65 | 0.1 | 5 | 0.016 | 0.01 | 0.015 | 0 | - | 0.20 | 0 | - |
| 127.0 | 1,371 | - | 2,742 | 0.320 | 0.27 | - | - | - | 2.29 | - | - |
| 16.0 | 134 | 7.1 | 17 | 0.020 | 0.02 | 0.037 | 0 | 0.007 | 0.15 | 0 | - |
| 8.4 | 74 | 0.8 | 30 | 0.020 | 0.02 | 0.043 | 0 | 0.010 | 0.15 | 0.76 | - |
| 22.5 | 233 | 1.5 | 435 | - | - | - | - | - | - | 49.50 | - |
| 46.0 | 385 | 2.9 | 1,144 | 0.160 | 0.06 | 0.090 | 0 | 0.010 | 0.57 | 105.00 | 0.58 |
| 18.0 | 242 | 4.6 | 153 | 0.080 | 0.05 | 0.120 | 0 | 0.010 | 0.46 | 6.12 | - |
| 32.0 | 277 | 4.8 | 160 | 0.080 | 0.05 | - | - | - | 0.48 | 6.40 | - |
| 26.0 | 220 | 8.0 | 140 | 0.080 | 0.02 | - | - | - | 0.40 | 4.0 | - |

# TABLE OF FOOD COMPOSITION

| FRUITS | Measure | Weight g | Calories | Protein g | Fats g | Carbohydrates g | Calcium mg | Iron mg | Magnesium mg |
|---|---|---|---|---|---|---|---|---|---|
| Lemon juice, fresh | 1 T | 15 | 4 | 0.1 | t | 1.2 | 1.0 | 0.03 | 4.5 |
| Nectarine, raw | 1 med | 87 | 50 | 0.5 | t | 12.0 | 3.1 | 0.39 | 11.3 |
| Olive, green, pickled | 1 lg | 7 | 9 | 0.1 | 0.9 | 0.1 | 4.3 | 0.11 | 1.54 |
| Olive, ripe, canned | 1 lg | 7 | 13 | 0.1 | 1.4 | 0.2 | 7.4 | 0.12 | - |
| Orange, fresh | 1 med | 180 | 88 | 1.8 | 0.4 | 20.0 | 74.0 | 0.72 | 19.8 |
| Papaya, raw | 1 lg | 400 | 156 | 2.4 | 0.4 | 40.0 | 80.0 | 1.20 | - |
| Peach, fresh | 1 med | 114 | 43 | 0.7 | 0.1 | 10.0 | 10.0 | 0.57 | 11.4 |
| Pears, fresh | 1 med | 182 | 111 | 1.3 | 0.7 | 27.8 | 15.0 | 0.60 | 12.7 |
| Persimmon, Japanese, raw | 1 med | 125 | 96 | 0.9 | 0.5 | 22.0 | 7.5 | 0.38 | 10.0 |
| Pineapple, raw | 1 cup | 140 | 73 | 0.5 | 0.3 | 17.0 | 24.0 | 0.70 | 17.0 |
| Plum, fresh, 2" Damson | 1 med | 60 | 29 | 0.3 | t | 6.7 | 7.2 | 0.30 | 5.4 |
| Prunes, dried, raw | 1 lg | 10 | 26 | 0.2 | 0.1 | 6.2 | 5.1 | 0.39 | 0.4 |
| Raisins, dried | 1 cup | 160 | 462 | 4.0 | 0.3 | 111.0 | 99.0 | 5.60 | 56.0 |
| Raspberries, red, raw | 1 cup | 133 | 76 | 1.6 | 0.7 | 16.0 | 29.0 | 1.20 | 26.6 |
| Strawberries, raw | 1 cup | 149 | 55 | 1.0 | 0.7 | 11.0 | 31.0 | 1.49 | 17.9 |
| Tangerine, raw | 1 lg | 114 | 52 | 0.9 | 0.2 | 12.0 | 46.0 | 0.46 | - |
| Watermelon, 4" x 8" piece | 1 wedge | 925 | 241 | 4.6 | 1.8 | 52.0 | 65.0 | 4.63 | 84.2 |

| Phosphorus mg | Potassium mg | Sodium mg | Vitamin A IU | (Thiamine) B$_1$ mg | (Riboflavin) B$_2$ mg | Vitamin B$_6$ mg | Vitamin B$_{12}$ mcg | Folic Acid mg | Niacin mg | Vitamin C mg | Vitamin E mg |
|---|---|---|---|---|---|---|---|---|---|---|---|
| 2.0 | 85 | 0.1 | 3 | 0.010 | t | 0.030 | - | t | 0.01 | 7.00 | - |
| 19.0 | 229 | 4.7 | 1,287 | t | t | 0.015 | 0 | 0.017 | - | 10.00 | - |
| 1.2 | 4 | 168.0 | 21 | 0 | 0 | - | 0 | - | - | t | - |
| 1.2 | 2 | 53.0 | 4.9 | t | t | 0.001 | 0 | t | - | - | - |
| 36.0 | 360 | 1.8 | 360 | 0.180 | 0.05 | 0.108 | 0 | 0.010 | 0.72 | 90.00 | 0.43 |
| 64.0 | 936 | 12.0 | 7,000 | 0.160 | 0.16 | - | 0 | - | 1.20 | 224.00 | - |
| 22.0 | 234 | 1.1 | 1,516 | 0.020 | 0.06 | 0.027 | 0 | 0.004 | 1.14 | 7.98 | - |
| 20.0 | 237 | 3.6 | 36 | 0.040 | 0.08 | 0.034 | 0 | - | 0.18 | 7.28 | - |
| 33.0 | 218 | 7.5 | 3,388 | 0.040 | 0.03 | - | - | - | 0.13 | 13.80 | - |
| 11.0 | 204 | 1.4 | 98 | 1.300 | 0.04 | 0.120 | 0 | 0.008 | 0.28 | 24.00 | - |
| 11.0 | 102 | 0.6 | 150 | 0.040 | 0.02 | 0.030 | 0 | - | 0.30 | 3.60 | - |
| 7.9 | 69 | 0.8 | 160 | 0.010 | 0.02 | 0.020 | 0 | 0.001 | 0.16 | 0.30 | - |
| 162.0 | 1,221 | 43.0 | 32 | 0.180 | 0.13 | 0.380 | 0 | 0.020 | 0.80 | 1.60 | - |
| 29.0 | 223 | 1.3 | 173 | 0.040 | 0.12 | 0.080 | 0 | 0.007 | 1.20 | 33.00 | - |
| 31.0 | 244 | 1.5 | 89 | 0.050 | 0.10 | 0.080 | 0 | 0.013 | 0.89 | 88.00 | 0.19 |
| 21.0 | 144 | 2.3 | 479 | 0.070 | 0.02 | 0.076 | 0 | 0.008 | 0.11 | 35.00 | - |
| 93.0 | 925 | 9.2 | 5,458 | 0.280 | 0.28 | 0.630 | 0 | 0.009 | 1.85 | 65.00 | |

# TABLE OF FOOD COMPOSITION

| NUTS, NUT PRODUCTS, AND SEEDS | Measure | Weight g | Calories | Protein g | Fats g | Carbohydrates g | Calcium mg | Iron mg | Magnesium mg |
|---|---|---|---|---|---|---|---|---|---|
| Almonds, dried | 1 cup | 140 | 765 | 26.0 | 76.0 | 26.0 | 328.0 | 6.58 | 378.0 |
| Brazil nuts, unsalted | 1 cup | 300 | 1,962 | 42.0 | 201.0 | 32.7 | 558.0 | 10.00 | 675.0 |
| Butternuts | 5 avg | 15 | 96 | 3.6 | 9.2 | 1.3 | - | 1.00 | - |
| Cashews, unsalted | 1 cup | 100 | 569 | 15.0 | 45.0 | 26.0 | 39.0 | 3.80 | 274.0 |
| Chestnuts, fresh | 1 cup | 200 | 382 | 5.8 | 3.0 | 84.2 | 54.0 | 3.40 | 82.0 |
| Coconut, fresh | 1 cup | 100 | 346 | 3.5 | 35.3 | 9.4 | 13.0 | 1.70 | 46.0 |
| Hazelnuts (filberts) | 11 avg | 15 | 97 | 1.6 | 9.5 | 3.0 | 38.0 | 0.50 | 27.6 |
| Hickory nuts | 15 sm | 15 | 101 | 2.1 | 10.1 | 2.0 | - | 0.40 | 24.0 |
| Peanuts, roasted, w/skin | 1 cup | 240 | 1,397 | 60.0 | 107.0 | 48.0 | 173.0 | 5.28 | 420.0 |
| Pistachio nuts | 1 cup | 100 | 594 | 19.0 | 54.0 | 19.0 | 131.0 | 7.30 | 158.0 |
| Pumpkin and Squash kernels | 1 cup | 230 | 1,271 | 67.0 | 107.0 | 35.0 | 117.0 | 26.00 | - |
| Sesame seeds, dry, decorticated | 1 cup | 230 | 1,339 | 42.0 | 123.0 | 41.0 | 253.0 | 5.50 | 416.0 |
| Sunflower seeds, dry | 1 cup | 100 | 560 | 24.0 | 43.0 | 19.0 | 120.0 | 7.10 | 38.0 |
| Walnuts, Black | 1 cup | 100 | 628 | 21.0 | 59.6 | 15.1 | t | 6.00 | 190.0 |
| Walnuts, English, raw | 1 cup | 100 | 651 | 15.0 | 59.0 | 15.0 | 99.0 | 3.10 | 131.0 |

| Phosphorus mg | Potassium mg | Sodium mg | Vitamin A IU | (Thiamine) $B_1$ mg | (Riboflavin) $B_2$ mg | Vitamin $B_6$ mg | Vitamin $B_{12}$ mcg | Folic Acid mg | Niacin mg | Vitamin C mg | Vitamin E mg |
|---|---|---|---|---|---|---|---|---|---|---|---|
| 706.0 | 1,082 | 5.6 | 0 | 0.340 | 1.29 | 0.140 | 0 | 0.063 | 4.90 | t | • |
| 2,088.0 | 2,145 | 3.0 | t | 3.300 | 0.36 | 0.510 | 0 | 0.015 | 4.60 | 30.00 | • |
| 373.0 | 464 | 15.0 | 100 | 0.430 | 0.25 | - | 0 | - | 1.80 | • | • |
| 176.0 | 908 | 12.0 | - | 0.440 | 0.44 | - | - | - | 0.12 | • | • |
| 95.0 | 256 | 23.0 | 0 | 0.050 | 0.02 | 0.044 | 0 | 0.028 | 0.50 | 3.00 | - |
| 48.0 | 71 | 0.1 | 16 | 0.069 | 0.08 | - | - | 0.010 | 0.80 | 1.10 | • |
| 54.0 | - | - | - | 0.080 | - | - | - | - | 0 | - | • |
| 976.0 | 1,683 | 12.0 | t | 0.770 | 0.32 | 0.700 | 0 | 0.140 | 40.00 | 2.40 | 18.50 |
| 500.0 | 972 | - | 230 | 0.670 | - | - | - | - | 1.40 | 0 | • |
| 2,631.0 | - | - | 161 | 0.550 | 0.44 | - | - | 5.50 | - | • | |
| 1,361.0 | - | - | - | 0.410 | 0.30 | • | • | - | 12.40 | 0 | - |
| 837.0 | 920 | 30.0 | 50 | 1.960 | 0.23 | • | • | - | 5.40 | • | • |
| 570.0 | 460 | 3.0 | 300 | 0.220 | 0.11 | - | - | 0.077 | 0.70 | • | • |
| 380.0 | 450 | 2.0 | 30 | 0.330 | 0.13 | 0.730 | 0 | 0.080 | 0.90 | 2 | |

# TABLE OF FOOD COMPOSITION

| VEGETABLES | Measure | Weight g | Calories | Protein g | Fats g | Carbohydrates g | Calcium mg | Iron mg | Magnesium mg |
|---|---|---|---|---|---|---|---|---|---|
| Artichoke, raw | 1 sm | 100 | 44 | 2.9 | 0.2 | 10.6 | 51.0 | 1.30 | - |
| Asparagus, raw | 1 spear | 16 | 4 | 0.4 | t | 0.8 | 3.5 | 1.60 | - |
| Beans, green, cooked | 1 cup | 125 | 31 | 2.0 | 0.2 | 8.9 | 62.5 | .75 | 40.0 |
| Beans, Lima, green, raw | 1 cup | 160 | 197 | 13.0 | 0.8 | 35.4 | 83.2 | 4.50 | 10.7 |
| Bean sproutes (mung beans) raw | 1 cup | 50 | - | 1.9 | 0.1 | 3.3 | 10.0 | 0.65 | - |
| Cabbage, shredded, raw | 1 cup | 105 | 25 | 1.4 | 0.2 | 5.7 | 51.5 | 0.42 | 14.0 |
| Cabbage, red, raw | 1 cup | 100 | 31 | 2.0 | 0.2 | 6.9 | 42.0 | 0.80 | 35.0 |
| Carrots, sliced, raw | 1 lg | 100 | 42 | 1.1 | 0.2 | 9.7 | 37.0 | 0.70 | 23.0 |
| Cauliflower, raw | 1 cup | 100 | 27 | 2.7 | 0.2 | 5.2 | 25.0 | 1.10 | 24.0 |
| Celery, stalk, raw | 1 lg | 50 | 8 | 0.4 | t | 2.0 | 0.2 | 0.15 | 11.0 |
| Chickpeas (garbanzos), dry, raw | ½ cup | 100 | 360 | 20.5 | 4.8 | 61.0 | 150.0 | 6.90 | - |
| Chives, chopped, raw | 1 T | 10 | 3 | 0.2 | t | 0.6 | 7.0 | 0.20 | - |
| Corn, on-the-cob, raw | 1 ear | 100 | 96 | 3.5 | 1.0 | 22.0 | 3.0 | 0.70 | 48.0 |
| Cucumber, raw, not pared | ½ med | 50 | 8 | 0.5 | t | 1.7 | 13.0 | 0.60 | 6.0 |
| Endive (escarole) raw | 1 cup | 228 | 46 | 3.9 | 0.2 | 9.3 | 17.8 | 39.00 | 22.8 |
| Garlic | 1 bulb | 2 | 2 | 0.1 | t | 0.6 | 0.6 | 0.03 | - |
| Kohlrabi, raw, sliced | 1 cup | 140 | 41 | 2.8 | 0.1 | 9.2 | 57.0 | 0.70 | 52.0 |
| Leeks, raw | 1 cup | 200 | 104 | 4.4 | 0.6 | 22.4 | 104.0 | 2.20 | 46.0 |
| Lettuce, Bibb, Boston | 3½ oz | 100 | 14 | 1.2 | 0.2 | 2.5 | 35.0 | 2.00 | - |
| Lettuce, Iceberg (head) | 3½ oz | 100 | 13 | 0.9 | 0.1 | 2.9 | 20.0 | 0.50 | 11.0 |

| Phosphorus mg | Potassium mg | Sodium mg | Vitamin A IU | (Thiamine) $B_1$ mg | (Riboflavin) $B_2$ mg | Vitamin $B_6$ mg | Vitamin $B_{12}$ mcg | Folic Acid mg | Niacin mg | Vitamin C mg | Vitamin E mg |
|---|---|---|---|---|---|---|---|---|---|---|---|
| 88.0 | 430 | 43.0 | 160 | 0.080 | 0.05 | - | - | - | 1.00 | 12.00 | - |
| 9.9 | 44 | 0.3 | 144 | 0.030 | 0.03 | 0.020 | - | 0.020 | 0.24 | 5.30 | - |
| 46.3 | 189 | 5.0 | 675 | 0.090 | 0.11 | 0.100 | 0 | 0.040 | 0.75 | 15.00 | - |
| 227.0 | 1,040 | 3.2 | 46.4 | 0.380 | 0.19 | 0.270 | - | 0.050 | 2.24 | 46.40 | - |
| 32.0 | 112 | 2.5 | 10 | 0.070 | 0.07 | - | - | - | 0.40 | 10.00 | - |
| 31.5 | 245 | 21.0 | 137 | 0.050 | 0.05 | 0.170 | 0 | 0.034 | 0.32 | 44.00 | - |
| - | 268 | 26.0 | 40 | 0.090 | 0.06 | - | - | - | 0.40 | 61.00 | - |
| 36.0 | 341 | 47.0 | 11,000 | 0.060 | 0.05 | 0.150 | 0 | 0.008 | 0.60 | 8.00 | 0.11 |
| 56.0 | 295 | 13.0 | 60 | 0.110 | 0.11 | 0.210 | 0 | 0.022 | 0.70 | 78.00 | - |
| 14.0 | 171 | 63.0 | 120 | 0.020 | 0.02 | 0.030 | 0 | 0.004 | 0.15 | 4.50 | 0.19 |
| 331.0 | 797 | 26.0 | 50 | 0.310 | 0.15 | 0.54 | - | 0.130 | 2.00 | - | - |
| 4.0 | 25 | - | 580 | 0.080 | 0.13 | - | - | - | 0.10 | 6.00 | - |
| 111.0 | 280 | - | 400 | .15 | 0.12 | - | - | - | 1.70 | 12.00 | - |
| 14.0 | 80 | 3.0 | 125 | 0.015 | 0.02 | 0.021 | 0 | 0.004 | 0.10 | 5.50 | - |
| 123.0 | 6,826 | 31.9 | 7,524 | 0.160 | 0.32 | 0.050 | 0 | 0.107 | 1.14 | 22.80 | - |
| 4.0 | 11 | 0.4 | t | 0.010 | t | - | - | - | 0.01 | 0.30 | - |
| 71.0 | 521 | 11.2 | 28 | 0.080 | 0.06 | - | - | - | 0.42 | 92.00 | - |
| 100.0 | 694 | 10.0 | 80 | 0.220 | 0.12 | - | - | - | 1.00 | 34.00 | 3.80 |
| 26.0 | 264 | 9.0 | 970 | 0.060 | 0.06 | - | - | - | 0.03 | 8.00 | - |
| 22.0 | 175 | 9.0 | 330 | 0.060 | 0.06 | 0.055 | 0 | 0.021 | 0.30 | 6.00 | 0.06 |

# TABLE OF FOOD COMPOSITION

| VEGETABLES | Measure | Weight g | Calories | Protein g | Fats g | Carbohydrates g | Calcium mg | Iron mg | Magnesium mg |
|---|---|---|---|---|---|---|---|---|---|
| Lettuce, leaf | 3½ oz | 100 | 18 | 1.3 | 0.3 | 3.5 | 68.0 | 1.40 | - |
| Lettuce, Romaine | 3½ oz | 100 | 18 | 1.3 | 0.3 | 3.5 | 68.0 | 1.40 | 11.0 |
| Onions, green, raw | 1 bulb | 8 | 4 | 0.1 | t | 0.8 | 3.2 | 0.05 | - |
| Parsley, chopped, raw | 1 cup | 56 | 25 | 2.0 | 0.3 | 4.8 | 114.0 | 3.50 | 23.0 |
| Peppers, sweet, green, raw | 1 lg | 100 | 22 | 1.2 | 0.2 | 4.8 | 9.0 | 0.70 | 18.0 |
| Potato, baked, w/skin | 1 med | 100 | 93 | 2.6 | 0.1 | 21.1 | 9.0 | 0.70 | 22.0 |
| Pumpkin, raw | ½ cup | 100 | 26 | 1.0 | 0.1 | 6.5 | 21.0 | 8.00 | 12.0 |
| Radish, raw, red | 1 sm | 10 | 2 | 0.1 | t | 0.4 | 3.0 | 0.10 | 1.5 |
| Rutabagas, raw | 1 cup | 150 | 69 | 1.6 | 1.5 | 16.5 | 99.0 | 0.60 | 22.5 |
| Spinach, raw | 1 cup | 100 | 26 | 3.2 | 0.3 | 4.3 | 93 | 3.10 | 88.0 |
| Squash, summer, raw | 1 cup | 200 | 38 | 2.2 | 0.2 | 8.4 | 56.0 | 0.80 | 32.0 |
| Squash, winter, boiled, mashed | 1 cup | 200 | 76 | 2.2 | 0.6 | 18.4 | 40.0 | 1.00 | 34.0 |
| Sweet potato, baked | 1 sm | 100 | 141 | 2.1 | 0.5 | 32.5 | 40.0 | 0.90 | 31.0 |
| Tomato, raw | 1 med | 150 | 33 | 1.6 | 0.3 | 7.1 | 19.5 | 0.75 | 21.0 |
| Turnip, raw | ½ cup | 100 | 30 | 1.0 | 0.2 | 6.6 | 39.0 | 0.50 | 20.0 |
| Turnip, tops, raw | 1 cup | 100 | 28 | 3.0 | 0.3 | 5.0 | 246.0 | 1.80 | 58.0 |
| Water chestnuts, Chinese, raw | 4 avg | 25 | 20 | 0.3 | t | 4.7 | 1.0 | 0.15 | - |
| Watercress | 1 cup | 50 | 10 | 1.1 | 0.1 | 1.5 | 75.5 | 0.85 | 10.0 |

| Phosphorus mg | Potassium mg | Sodium mg | Vitamin A IU | (Thiamine) B$_1$ mg | (Riboflavin) B$_2$ mg | Vitamin B$_6$ mg | Vitamin B$_{12}$ mcg | Folic Acid mg | Niacin mg | Vitamin C mg | Vitamin E mg |
|---|---|---|---|---|---|---|---|---|---|---|---|
| 25.0 | 264 | 9.0 | 1,900 | 0.050 | 0.08 | - | - | 0.044 | 0.40 | 18.00 | - |
| 25.0 | 264 | 9.0 | 1,900 | 0.050 | 0.08 | - | - | - | 0.40 | 18.00 | - |
| 3.1 | 18 | 0.4 | t | 0.004 | t | - | 0 | 0.001 | 0.03 | 2.00 | - |
| 35.3 | 407 | 25.0 | 4,760 | 0.070 | 0.11 | 0.090 | 0 | 0.020 | 0.67 | 96.30 | 3.10 |
| 22.0 | 213 | 13.0 | 420 | 0.080 | 0.08 | 0.260 | 0 | 0.007 | 0.50 | 128.00 | - |
| 65.0 | 503 | 4.0 | t | 0.100 | 0.04 | 0.233 | - | - | 1.70 | 20.00 | 0.03 |
| 44.0 | 340 | 1.0 | 1,600 | 0.050 | 0.11 | - | - | - | 0.60 | 9.00 | |
| 3.1 | 32 | 1.8 | 1 | 0.003 | t | t | 0 | 0.001 | 0.03 | 2.60 | - |
| 58.5 | 360 | 7.5 | 870 | 0.110 | 0.11 | - | - | - | 1.60 | 64.30 | - |
| 51.0 | 470 | 71.0 | 8,100 | 0.100 | 0.20 | - | - | - | 0.60 | 51.00 | • |
| 58.0 | 404 | 2.0 | 820 | 0.100 | 0.18 | 0.126 | - | 0.034 | 2.00 | 44.00 | - |
| 64.0 | 516 | 2.0 | 7,000 | 0.080 | 0.20 | 0.182 | 0 | 0.024 | 0.80 | 16.00 | - |
| 58.0 | 300 | 12.0 | 8,100 | 0.090 | 0.07 | 0.218 | 0 | 0.015 | 0.70 | 22.00 | - |
| 40.5 | 366 | 1.5 | 1,390 | 0.090 | 0.06 | 0.150 | 0 | 0.012 | 1.95 | 34.50 | 0.60 |
| 30.0 | 268 | 49.0 | - | 0.040 | 0.07 | - | - | - | 0.60 | 36.00 | - |
| 58.0 | 312 | - | 7,600 | 0.210 | 0.39 | - | - | - | 0.80 | 139.00 | • |
| 16.3 | 125 | 5.0 | 0 | 0.040 | 0.05 | - | - | - | 0.25 | 1.00 | - |
| 27.0 | 141 | 21.0 | 2,450 | 0.040 | 0.08 | - | - | - | 0.45 | 39.50 | |

# MOST DANGEROUS FOOD ADDITIVES

| Chemicals | Used as | Danger | Foods with These Additives |
|---|---|---|---|
| **BHA** (butylated hydroxyanisole) **BHT** (butylated hydroxytoluene) | Preservative | May cause cancer, liver problems | Vegetable oils, many dry cereals, frozen pizzas, fresh pork and pork sausage, potato chips, drink powders, punches, doughnuts, shortenings, steak sauces, vegetables packed with sauces, breakfast drinks, potatoes (packaged), nuts, canned puddings, toaster tarts, dry soup mixes, crackers, gelatin desserts, dry yeast, instant teas. |
| **CAFFEINE** | Coloring, flavoring | Can cause nervousness, heart palpitations; suspect as causing birth defects; known to be stimulant and diuretic. | Naturally occurring in coffee, tea, cocoa; put in bakery goods and soft drinks. |
| **CARRA-GEENAN** | Thickener. Binds food particles together. | Indicated in colon disorders. Study indicates possible intestinal ulcer causative. FDA suspects possible genetic effects. | Ice cream, beer, sour cream, baby formulas, yogurt, jelly, cookie dough, evaporated milk, cottage cheese, whipped toppings, punch drinks, bread, olives, chocolate milk, vegetables packaged with sauces, gelatin and pudding desserts. |

| | Use | Effects | Found in |
|---|---|---|---|
| **MODIFIED FOOD STARCH** | Cheap filler in foods. A thickening agent. | Sodium hydroxide in it may cause lung damage, vomiting. FDA plans further study. | Soups, gravies, baked beans, beets canned in jars, cream style canned corn, dry-roasted nuts, drink powders, ravioli, baby foods, frozen pizzas, pie fillings, frozen fish (packaged), baking powder. |
| **MSG** (monosodium glutamate) | Flavoring. | May cause chilling, sweating, headaches, chest pains. Cause possibly of birth defects has prompted FDA to intensive study. Not used in baby foods since 1969. | Processed cheeses, salad dressings, dry roasted nuts, soup mixes, canned soups, beer, frozen pizzas, broths, Chinese foods, vegetables packaged with sauce, canned meats, packaged sea foods, frankfurters, tomato paste, meat tenderizers, bread crumbs, croutons. |
| **NITRITES, SODIUM NITRATES, SODIUM** | Preservative. Coloring. Curing. | Poison overdoses have been fatal. Combine with other chemicals in body to form cancer causing substances. Prohibited in fish in Canada. May have reproduction consequences. FDA studying. | Sausages, smoked fish, baby foods, bacon, smoked and processed meats (salami, tongue, ham, corned beef, pastrami), frozen pizzas. |
| **RED DYE 40** (Allura Red AC) | Coloring | Possible cancer causative. May cause birth defects. FDA investigating. | Gelatin desserts, chewing gum, red pistachios, cereals, baked goods, soft drinks, candies. |

| SACCHARIN | Sugar substitute. Sweetener for diabetics. Low calorie sweetener. | May cause bladder cancer, tumors. Causes allergic reaction affecting skin, heartbeat, gastro-intestinal disorders. | Breakfast drinks, plain and diet sodas, gingerale and as sweetener (sugar substitute in many diet foods and products). |
| SODIUM ERYTHORBATE | Coloring. Freshener. Preservative. | May be factor in genetic effects. Banned in some countries. | Ham, turkey roast (frozen), baked goods, bacon, frankfurters, potato salad, beverages. |

# CONVENIENT EQUIVALENTS CHART

| Food | Amount | Approximate Yield |
|------|--------|-------------------|
| Butter | 4 oz. | ½ C. (1 stick) |
| Carob, powdered | 1 oz. | 5 T. |
| chips | 6 oz. | 1 C. |
| Coconut, shredded | 4 oz. | 1⅓ C. |
| Coffee, ground | 1 lb. | 80 T. |
| Corn meal | 1 lb. | 3 C. |
| Cream, whipping | 8 oz. | 1 C. |
| Eggs, whole | 5 | 1 C. |
| whites | 8-10 | 1 C. |
| yolks | 12-15 | 1 C. |
| Flour, whole wheat | 1 lb. | 4 C. |
| Buckwheat | 1 lb. | 4 C. |
| Honey | ¾ lb. | 1 C. |
| Lemon, medium | 1 | 3 T. juice & 2 t. grated rind |
| Noodles | 1 lb. | 3½ to 4 C. |
| Nuts, shelled | 1 lb. | 3½ to 4 C. |
| Onion, medium | 1 | ½ C. chopped |
| Orange, medium | 1 | ⅓ C. juice & 1 T. grated rind |
| Raisins | 1 lb. | 2½ C. |
| Rice, uncooked, long grain | 1 C. | 4 C. cooked |
| Spaghetti | 4 oz. | 2 C. cooked |
| Sugar, raw | 1 lb. | 2¼ C. firm-packed |
| date | ¼ lb. | 1 C. |
| Yeast, dry | 1 oz. | 4 T. |

## STANDARD ABBREVIATIONS

t.   = teaspoon

T.   = tablespoon

C.   = cup

gm.  = gram

mg.  = milligram

oz.  = ounce

lb.  = pound

## EQUIVALENT MEASURES

Dash or pinch = less
than ⅛ teaspoon

3 teaspoons = 1 tablespoon

4 tablespoons = ¼ cup =
2 ounces

8 tablespoons = ½ cup =
4 ounces

2 cups = 1 pint

2 pints = 1 quart

4 quarts = 1 gallon

# SOURCE DIRECTORY OF PRODUCTS AND SERVICES

We have no connection with, nor do we receive any financial compensation from, any of the companies noted below. They are simply listed here to aid readers in their search for better health.

**APHRODISIA**, 28 Carmine St., New York, NY 10014. Alfalfa, fenugreek, flax, black and yellow mustard seeds, safflower, sesame seeds. Catalog.

**BEALE'S FAMOUS PRODUCTS**, Box 323, Ft. Washington, PA 19034. Unglazed pottery sprouter, assortment of 15 different seeds, breakfast mix, salad mix, sandwich mix, books. Send for price lists.

**BRONSON PHARMACEUTICALS**, 4526 Rinetti Lane, LaCanada, CA 91011. For vitamin C crystals as Ascorbic Acid, Sodium Ascorbate, Calcium Ascorbate, etc.

**D. V. BURRELL SEED GROWERS CO.**, P.O. Box 150, Rockey Ford, CO 81067.

**CHAMPLAIN VALLEY SEEDS**, Box 454, Westport, NY 12993. Buckwheat.

**CROSS SEED CO.**, Route 1, Box 125, Bunker Hill, KS 67676. Alfalfa, wheat, rye.

**DIAMOND K ENTERPRISES**, St. Charles, MN 55972. (507-932-4308) Sunflower seed. Request black ones used in oil making.

**FRAZIER FARMS**, 11655 Duenda Rd., Rancho Bernardo, CA 92128. Write for price lists for seeds, raw carob, agar, etc.

**JUICE SUITE**, P.O. Box 701, Bloomfield, CT 06002. Grass juicers, distillers, blenders and vegetable juicers. Discount on many of the appliances. Send 50¢ for information and price lists.

**LIVING FARMS**, 200 3rd St., Tracy, MN 56175. Alfalfa, wheat, rye and red clover.

**MIXMASTER**, with attachments. Available at department, hardware and health food stores.

**MOULINEX**, made in France. A nut, spice and coffee grinder typically available in health food stores.

**NATURAL DEVELOPMENT CO.**, Bainbridge, PA 17502. Cress seeds, sunflower seeds, buckwheat, lentils, corn, wheat, alfalfa. Free postage east of the Mississippi River. Free catalog.

**NUTRI-FLOW,** 2123 S.W. Camelot Court, Portland, OR 97225. Food dehydrator manufacturer.

**L. L. OLDS SEED CO.**, 2901 Packers Avenue, P.O. Box 1069, Madison, WI 53701.

**ORGANIC FARM AND GARDEN CENTER,** Box 2806, San Rafael, CA 94901.

**PLASTAKET MANUFACTURING INC.**, 6226 Highway 12, Lodi, CA 95240. Manufacturers of the Champion food processor.

**THE REBOUNDER,** Olympus Distributing Corp., P.O. Box 969, St. George, UT 84770. (801-673-3005) Circular trampoline ideal for all kinds of aerobic exercises.

**RELIANCE PRODUCTS,** 1900 Olympic Blvd., Walnut Creek, CA 94596. Request catalog: Storage/Survival foods, independent/self-sufficient living; outdoor enjoyment; kitchen/food machine.

**RIGGSCRAFT,** P.O. Box 1273, Laramie, WY 82070. Shippers of sprout-quality seeds, beans and grains. Free catalog.

**SHILOH FARMS,** Route 59, Sulphur Springs, AR 72768. Ask for price list (seeds, foods).

**SUNDANCE INDUSTRIES,** 28 Vermont Avenue, White Plains, NY 10606. (914-946-9340) Their Wheatena model "S" is an ideal juicer for wheat grass and sprouted grains.

**VITA MIX CORP.**, 8615 Usher Road, Cleveland, OH 44138. (216-235-4840) Their model 3600 is an excellent blender and grain and seed grinder.

**WALNUT ACRES,** Penns Creek, PA 17862. Grains, seeds, granolas; lots of natural foods, kitchen appliances and equipment. Catalog.

# Glossary

**Agar-Agar**
a gelatinous extract (dried) from sea algae used as congealant and thickener. Rich in minerals.

**Amaranth**
ancient seed-yielding plant native to many areas of world, especially Mexico. Used for flour and a confection (Mex.). Highly nutritious.

**Arrowroot**
a tropical American root plant yielding nutritious starch. Used in powder form as a thickener.

**Ascorbic Acid**
(fine crystals)
Vitamin C. An efficacious food supplement, flavor enhancer and food stabilizer.

**Barley Malt**
(syrup and powder)
a nutritious food sweetener used as alternative to sugar. Made from sweet barley.

**Carob**
a Mediterranean tree yielding sweet pods with taste similar to cocoa. Sold as toasted or raw powder. Contains B vitamins and carbohydrates. The nutritious food St. John lived on.

**Chia**
the seed of a plant native to America. Highly nutritious. Energy and endurance food of American Indians. Used as condiment, for sprouting and medicinally.

**Cold Pressed Oil**
vegetable oils that have been extracted from seeds by a method that does not heat the oil too high with damaging and nutrient-destroying temperatures.

**Comfrey**
a large-leaf, blue-flowered, tuberous-root plant of the borage family.

Used medicinally for salads and green drinks. Highly nutritious. Contains vitamin B12. Cultivation encouraged by world organizations for famine relief. Good source of magnesium.

Dulse
a tasty sea lettuce twelve times more nutritious than the average vegetable. Sold in dehydrated form or powder. Used as condiment in salads, casseroles, breads, etc.

Fenugreek
a leguminous Asiatic herb used in curries and for sprouting. Extremely high in vitamin B3.

Flaxseed
a seed of the flax (linen) plant. Used for oil (highest in vitamin E of any seed known), for seed "cheeses" and dressings, as a thickener and medicinally as a demulcent and emollient.

Jícama
South American root vegetable. Its juicy crispness and mild flavor make it a favorite. Imported from Mexico. (Pronounced *hee*-kah-mah)

Kelp
a sea plant with full complement of naturally chelated minerals. Sold in powder or granular form. Used as supplement in mineral deficiencies, as aid in losing weight and as salt substitute.

Lecithin
an oil-like product of soy beans. Sold as liquid or granules. Used as food stabilizer and medicinally.

Miso
a paste-like, fermented product of soy. Used in salad sauces, dips, etc.

Molasses
the thick dark syrup separated from raw sugar in the manufacture of sugar. Rich in minerals.

Piloncillo (Mex.) or Panela (S. Amer.)
a dark, hard brick or cone of molasses crystals separated out in the process of sugar refining. Rich in minerals.

Poi
an Oriental, high quality starch food served with fish.

Pollen, or Bee Pollen
the flower pollen collected on the hind legs of bees. It is a complete food, rich in B vitamins.

Rice Bran
> the outer, golden-colored hull from whole grain rice. Used in breads, cakes, cereals. Highly nutritious in B vitamins, especially vitamin B$_1$.

Rich Polish
> the inner part of the hull that is polished off rice grains to produce white rice. A good source of B vitamins, some minerals and protein.

Rice Syrup
> a nutritious sweetener made from sweet rice.

Sodium Ascorbate
(powder)
> a common form of vitamin C. An effective food supplement, salt substitute and food stabilizer.

Spirulina Plankton
> a fresh-water algae harvested in alkaline lakes as Lake Texcoco near Mexico City, or Lake Chad in Africa, or man-made tanks in California, Japan, Korea, etc. A complete food, known for its high protein, vitamin B$_{12}$ and chlorophyl content. An excellent supplement for deficiencies.

Tamari
> a fermented, aged product made from soy. Used as sauce and condiment in sauces, on rice, etc. Nutritious and flavorful. Similar to soy sauce but less salty.

Tofu
> a mild curd made from soy milk. Used as cow milk cheese alternate.

Torula Yeast
> a nutritional yeast cultured on wood pulp. Does not contain selenium. High in B vitamins.

Triticale
> a cereal grain resulting from cross pollination of wheat and rye. Reportedly higher in protein than either parent grain, it resembles wheat.

Vanilla Bean Pod
> the pod and bean of some tropical American vine orchids from which vanilla extract is made. Used for flavoring and, rubbed on skin, as perfume.

Yeast, Primary Brewer's
> a fungus or yeast cultured on molasses. Used as nutritional food supplement. High in B vitamins and minerals, especially selenium. A complete food except for vitamin C.

# BIBLIOGRAPHY

AIROLA, PAAVO
*How to Get Well.*
*How to Stay Slim, Healthy and Young With Juice Fasting.*
Phoenix, Az: Health Plus Publishers, P. O. Box 22001 -
85028.

BAKER, ELIZABETH AND DR. ELTON.
*The Uncook Book.* *1981.*
*The Unmedical Book.* *1988.*
*The Unmedical Miracle-Oxygen.* Indianola, WA; Drelwood
Communications, P. O. Box 149 - 98342. 1991.

BUCKINGER, OTTO H. F.
*About Fasting--A Royal Road to Healing.* Wellingborough,
Northamptonshire: Thorsons Publishers Limited, 1976.

CARTER, ALBERT E.
*The Miracles of Rebound Exercise.* Bothell, WA: The
National Institute of Reboundology & Health, Inc., 1979.

DIAMOND, JOHN.
*Your Body Doesn't Lie.* New York, NY: Warner Books, Inc.,
1979.

FREDERICKS, CARLTON.
*Psycho-Nutrition.* New York, NY: Grosset & Dunlap, A
Filmways Company Publishers, 1978.

GERRAS, CHARLES, Editor.
*Feasting On Raw Foods.* Emmaus, PA: Rodale Press, 1980.

GRAY, ROBERT.
*The Colon Clensing Handbook.* Oakland, CA: Rockbridge
Publishing Co., 1982.

KLINE, MONTE L. AND STRUBE, W. P., Jr.
*Eat, Drink and Be Ready.* Fort Worth, TX: Harvest Press,
Inc., 1977.

KULVINSKAS, VIKTORAS.
*Sprouts For the Love of Every Body.* Wethersfield, CT:
Omango D'Press, 1978.

LESSER, MICHAEL, M. D.
*Nutrition and Vitamin Therapy.* New York, NY: Random
House Gross Press, Inc.

LOVETT, C. S.
*Help, Lord, The Devil Wants Me Fat.* Personal
Christianity, Baldwin Park, CA. 91706

MUNROE, ESTHER.
*Sprouts To Grow And Eat*.    Brattleboro, VT: The Stephen Green Press, 1977.

PAULING, LINUS.
*Vitamin C, the Common Cold, And The Flu*. San Francisco, CA: W. H. Freeman and Company, 1976.

PFEIFFER, CARL C.
*Mental And Elemental Nutrients*. New Canaan, CT: Keats Publishing, Inc., 1975.

THOMSEN, M. D.
*Medical Wisdom From The Bible*. (Spire Books); Fleming H. Revell Co., Old Tappan, NJ 07675.

TAYLOR, RENEE
*Come Along to Hunza*. Minneapolis, Minn. 55401. Dennison and Co. Inc.

WHYTE, KAREN CROSS
*The Complete Sprouting Cookbook*.    San Franciso, CA; Troubador Press, 1973.

WIGMORE, ANN.
*Be Your Own Doctor*. New York, NY: Hemisphere Press.

WILLIAMS, ROGER J.
*Nutrition Against Disease*. New York, NY: Bantam Books, 1973.

# Index

## A

Abbreviations of measurements, 15, 194
Additives, most dangerous, 15, 190-93
Allergies, 45, 56, 107-10, 114, 117
Almond butter dressing, 153
Almond paste tacos, 37
Amaranth stove-top muffins, 149
Apple crisp, 24
Apple jam, 97
Apple sauce cake, 49
Arthritis, 104, 110, 115, 117
Asthma, 56
Atherosclerosis, 45, 123
Avocado paste, 48

## B

Banana fruit cake, 47
Barley pancakes, 36
Barley stove-top muffins #2, 50
Barley-vegetable soup, 62
Basic pie crust, 165
Basic whole grain bread, 147
Basic whole grain crackers, 148
Bean soup-of-the-day, 81
Beef noodle stew, 83
Bee pollen, 124
Beet soup, 151
Berry-date syrup, 23

Bible quotations; Corinthians 6:19 & 20 - 53;
    Ezekiel 47:12 - 119; Genesis 1.11 - 146;
    Genesis 1:29 - 11; Genesis 1.29 - 90;
    Genesis 2:9 - 15; Genesis 6:21 - 123;
    Genesis 41:35 - 139; III John 2 - 27;
    Leviticus 11:47 - 41; Philippians 2:13 -
    127; Proverbs 3:18 & 19 - 75; Proverbs
    10:5 - 131; Proverbs 17:22 - 143; Prov-
    erbs 22:9 - 65; Proverbs 23:6 - 107;
    Proverbs 24:13 & 14 - 87; Revelations
    2:22 - 11, 90; Romans 8:28 - 143
Birthday fruit cake, 159
Birth defects, 114
Blackberry ice cream, 162
Blueberry- buckwheat (or raisin) muffins, 23
Blueberry ice cream, 163
Bran muffins, 20
Breakfast cake, 161
Brown beans, 58
Brown rice casserole, 59
Brown roast soup, 51
Buckwheat crackers, 95
Buckwheat pancakes, 46
Buckwheat stove-top muffins, 33
Budded, buttered seeds, 60
Budded sunflower seeds, 46
Buttered beets, 38
Buttered buckwheat crunchies, 63
Buttered peas, fresh or frozen, 70
Butter malt syrup, 36

## C

Cabbage-pineapple salad, 99
Caffeine, 177, *see also* coffee
Cancer, 104, 115, 135
Cantaloupe seed milk shake, 97
Carbohydrates: in starches, 120; in fruits, 120
Carbonated drinks, 117
Caroban pudding, 59
Carob cake, 158
Carob chip topping, 159
Carrot cake, 38, 160
Cataracts, 56
Celery soup, 152
Cereals: 156
    granola, 156; granola gold, 81; oatmeal sunflower, 34; oatmeal supreme, 80; sprout cereal, 156; sprouted oat, 84; sprouted rye, 71
Cereal topping, 83
Chemotherapy sickness remedy, 123-24
Chicken dumplings, 73
Chicken production, 115
Chilled cream-of-corn soup, 70
Chinese chicken with vegies, 82
Cinnamon carob tea, 37
Clarity of thinking, 143
Coffee, getting off of, 75-77
Colitis, 56
Colon: cleansing of, 104-06; problems from milk products, 116
Comfrey spice tea, 35
Complete person, the, 11, 12
Cornmeal mush-with-a-flair, 59
Cornsilk tea, 84
Corn stove-top muffins, 35
Constipation, 104, 116
Cookies, *see* desserts, sweet treats
Creamed dried beef, 34

## D

Dehydrating foods: 139-41
    added benefits of, 140-41; commercial or hand made dryers, 140; oven drying, 140; sun drying, 139
Daily menus, 16-18, 27-30, 41-44, 53-56, 65-68, 75-77, 87-90
Dairy products: *see* milk
Date butterscotch pie, 51
Date darko, 70
Date jam, 20
Date whip, 21

Desserts, sweet treats:
    apple sauce cake, 49; banana fruit cake, 47; caroban pudding, 59; carrot cake, 38; date butterscotch pie, 51; date darko, 70; frozen bananas, 48; fruit granola bars, 73; granola bars, 92; oatmeal coconut cookies, 35; oatmeal fig cookies, 80; pear cake, 71; pecan pie, 61; prune parfait, 72; prune whip, 22; raisin sesame circles, 72; rice cookies, 25
Diabetes, 104, 123
Digestive system, cleaning of, 103-06
Dried apple jam, 31
Dulse, 125

## E

Eden corn, 32
Eggs on buckwheat crunchies, 98
Eggs on oatmeal, 93
Enema taking, 104-05, 106
Equivalents, convenient chart of, 193-94
Essene wheat bread, 96
Exercises, 19-20, 30-31, 45-46, 56-57, 69, 78-79, 91-92
Eye problems, 104

## F

Fats: natural oils and fats, 121; processed oils, 27-30, 30
Fiber, in diet, 104
Fig jam, 23
Fish, 115
Fish-rice casserole, 79
Flaxseed dressing, 98, 153
Food composition, table of: in fruits, 180-83; in nuts and seeds, 184-85; in vegetables, 186-89
Fresh gumbo soup, 152
Fresh vegetable stew, 96
Frozen bananas, 48
Fruit-granola bars, 85
Fruit salad dressing, 71

## G

Gardening indoors, 68, 131-35
harvesting of foods, 135; list of needed equipment, 131-32; planting seeds, 134; preparing soil, 133; seeds and grain sources, 132-33; sprouting chart, 136-37
God, 11, 19, 56, 68, 90-91, 113, 117, 122, 123, 135, 143, 144
Granola, 156
Granola bars and cookies, 92, 156-58, *see also* desserts
Granola gold, 81
Green drinks, 166-67
Guacamole, 39
Guacamole dip, 85
Guacamole dressing, 152

## H

Harmful ingredients (artificial colors, flavors, preservatives), 114, 117
Heart trouble, 104
Heavenly fresh apple pie, 166
Heavenly fruit pies and crusts, 164-66; basic pie crust, 165; heavenly fresh apple pie, 165; heavenly raw apricot pie, 165; *see also* desserts
Heavenly raw apricot pie, 165
Helpful hints, 167-68
Honey butter, 21
Honey glazed parsnips or carrots, 48
Hot chocarob, 21
Hypoglycemia, 104

## I

Ice creams: 161-64
blackberry, 162; blueberry, 163; peach, 162; tart apple, 162; unique berry, 163; unique orange-apricot, 164
Indoor gardening, *see* gardening indoors

## J

Jams, 20, 22, 23, 31, 49, 50, 97

## K

Kelp, 124
Kitchen equipment: 15, 127-29
blender, 128; grinder, 128; juicer, 128-29; knives, 127; seed mill, 128
Kinesiology testing, 106, 107-11

## L

Lemon butter sauce, 32
Lemon butter sauce for salmon, 84
Lemon grass tea, 33
Lentil soup, 48

## M

Macaroni with cheese, 36
Mashed potatoes supreme, 69
Meat, 115
Meat loaf, 63
Mental retardation, 114
Mexican scrambled egg or omelet, 79
Milk: getting off of, 53-56; hazards in, 115-16
Millet stove-top muffins, 57
Millet vegetable casserole, 47
Minerals: 173-79
calcium, 173; chlorine, 173; chromium, 173-74; cobalt, 174; copper, 174; fluorine, 174; iodine, 174; iron, 175; lithium, 175; magnesium, 175; manganese, 176; molybdenum, 176; phosphorus, 176-77; potassium, 177; selenium, 177; silicon, 177; sodium, 178; sulfur, 178; zinc, 178-79
Mock-tuna on rye, 80
Molasses, 125
Morning sickness remedy, 123-24

## N

Natural food alternatives: 68, 90-91, 119-22; carbohydrates (in fruits and starches), 120; dark green leafy vegetables, 121; herbal teas, 121; oils and fats, 121; proteins in animal products, 120; proteins in plants, 119; seasoning and condiments, 121; sweeteners, 121
Nut butter, 24
Nut butter sandwich, 94
Nutmeat loaf or patties, 150
Nut meat patties, 94

## O

Oatmeal coconut cookies, 35
Oatmeal fig cookies, 80
Oatmeal-sunflower cereal, 34
Oatmeal supreme, 80
Oil and vinegar dressing, 154
Orange cake, 160

## P

Papaya seed pepper, 51
Peach Ice Cream, 162
Peanut butter pocket bread, 21
Pear cake, 71
Pecan butter, 98
Pecan pie, 61
Pizza crust, cooked, 150; raw, 151
Poached salmon, 83
Primary yeast, 123-24
Processed foods: getting off of, 65-68, 104; hazards of, 113-18
Proteins: in animal products, 120; in plants, 119
Prune parfait, 72
Prune whip, 22

## R

Rabbit noodle casserole, 50
Raisin-bran muffins, 61
Raisin jam, 22, 50
Raisin-sesame circles, 72
Raw applesauce, 58
Raw sprouted grain crackers, 149
Raw tomato sauce, 73
Recipe notes in a nutshell, 167-68
Red clover-fruit tea, 93
Rice bran stove-top muffins, 62
Rice cake-peanut butter munchies, 34
Rice cookies, 25
Rice casserole with chopped beef, 22
Roast lamb or roast beef, 51
Romaine tacos, 82
Royal jelly, 124, 125

## S

Salads:
    cabbage-pineapple, 99; creative salad combinations, 154-55; salad sprouts, 155; spinach, 33; sprout garden salad, 95; tomato-cucumber, 22; waldorf, 14
Salad dressings: 152-54
    almond butter, 153; flaxseed, 98, 153; fruit salad, 71; guacamole, 152; oil and vinegar, 154; sesame seed, 153; sunflower, 153; tomato purée, 154
Salad tacos, 31
Salmon croquettes, 84
Seasonings and condiments, 121, 140, 141
Seed meat loaf or patties, 150
Seed and nut meat loaves, patties and pizza, 149-51; nut meat loaf or patties, 150; nut meat patties, 94; pizza crust, cooked, 150; pizza crust, raw, 151; seed meat loaf or patties, 150; vegetarian pizza filling, 151
Sesame seed cheese, 95
Sesame seed dressing, 153
Sesame seed spread, 58
Sesame-sunflower seed dip, 99
Sinus trouble, 56
Soaked almonds, 46
Soft scrambled eggs, 60
Soups, cooked and raw: 151-52
    barley-vegetable, 62; bean, 81; beet, 151; brown roast, 51; celery, 152; chilled cream of corn, 70; fresh gumbo, 152; lentil, 48; sprouted lentil, 38; tomato, 152; yellow squash with mushrooms, 94
Sources of products and services, 195-96
Southern spoon bread, 72
Special foods shopping list, 15, 27, 41, 53, 65, 75, 87
Spinach salad, 33
Spirulina plankton, 123
Sprout cereal, 156
Sprouted lentil soup, 38
Sprouted oat cereal, 84
Sprouted rye cereal, 71
Sprout garden salad, 95
Sprouting, 87, 131-35; chart, 136-37; for salads, 155
Stable emotions, 143-44
Strawberry jam, 49
Sugar, dangers of, 113-14; getting off of, 16-18, 18-19; in history, 114, 123; substitutes, 18-19, 121
Sunflower seed dressing, 153
Supplements, natural food, 123-25
Sweeteners, 121

## T

Tart apple ice cream, 162
Teas, 18-19, 33, 35, 37, 78, 84, 93, 105,
    121-22, 140, 166
Temperance, 144
Thickening agents, 164
Tomato-cucumber salad, 22
Tomato purée dressing, 154
Tomato soup, 152
Toxic substances, 107-08, 109, 114, 140,
    147
Traditional diet, 103

## U

Unique berry ice cream, 163
Unique orange-apricot ice cream, 164

## V

Vegetables, dark green leafy, 121
Vegetarian pizza filling, 151
Vegetable plate, 60
Vitamins, 169-73
    A, 169-70; B complex, 170; C, 170-
    71; D, 171; E, 171-72; F, 172; G, 172;
    K, 172; T, 172-73

## W

Waldorf salad, 14
Watermelon breakfast, 92
Wheat, 117
Wheatgrass, 135
Wheat milk, 81
White flour, getting off of, 41-45; hazards of,
    114, 123
Whole grain breads and crackers, 147-49
    Amaranth stove-top muffins, 149; basic
    sprouted grain crackers, 148; basic whole
    grain bread, 147; basic whole grain
    crackers, 148; raw sprouted grain
    crackers, 149
    149
Whole grain cakes, 158-61
    breakfast cake, 161; birthday fruit cake,
    129; carob cake, 158; carob chip top-
    ping, 159; carrot cake, 160; orange
    cake, 160; see also desserts

## Y

Yam sticks, 37
Yellow squash soup with mushrooms, 94

## IN APPRECIATION

I first met Elizabeth and Dr. Elton Baker at a convention of the National Health Federation where we had all just lectured. I found the Bakers to be a charming, articulate couple, extremely knowledgeable about nutrition. I was also impressed with their comprehension of the Bible, the word of God. They have the ability to take the wisdom of the Scriptures and apply it to nutrition.

They gave me a copy of their first work, THE UNCOOK BOOK. Since that time I have had the opportunity to read it, an experience that fortified my first impression of this remarkable couple.

Shortly after our meeting, Elizabeth telephoned saying she and Dr. Baker were finishing a new book and asked if I would consider writing a forward for it. I told her I would be happy to look at the manuscript.

At first glance it appeared to be primarily a book of menus and recipes. What bothered me, however, was a seeming lack of good nutritional practice. There was a complete deficiency of appreciation for the Metabolic diet, which has proven so successful in the prevention and treatment of diseases such as cancer, arthritis and multiple sclerosis.

While scanning through I shuddered when bacon and eggs were suggested for breakfast. Another breakfast had sausages. Still another contained English muffins. Dinners consisted of such things as roast pork and white rice casseroles. Certainly with a diet such as this, I could hardly write a foreword endorsing this book! What concerned me even more was that I could not believe this was written by the same enlightened couple I had recently met.

Before sending it back with a note of refusal, I felt I owed it to them to go over it more thoroughly. As I read it carefully this time, I became engrossed. I realized that my original evaluation of the Bakers was correct; not only were they knowledgeable nutritionists, but nutritional geniuses! They had come up with a solution to the problems all Metabolic Therapists have in giving their patients a natural foods diet.

Most patients cannot make the transition from a "junk food" diet to a natural one. As a result, they continue to stay on their old foods and hope that the pills alone will do the work of restoring their health. Elizabeth and Elton realized this and felt that the only way to make the transition was gradually. They actually

do it in seven phases.  The first phase is conventional:
bacon, sausage, English muffins, white rice, etc.  It is
a starting place.  Anyone can follow the menus in the
first phase.  As the reader progresses to each successive
phase, he or she becomes more intensely involved with
natural foods.  It is done in such a beautiful way that
the transition is easy to make.

As each phase is introduced, not only are the menus
give, but also complete recipes.  This innovative,
pioneering approach to nutrition is enough to make THE
UN-DIET BOOK one of the more important books to come
along in some time.  But they don't stop there.

The human body contains three parts.  It is
physical, mental and spiritual.  All parts must be kept
healthy if we are to live a full, disease-free life.  In
addition to the menus and recipes, each phase is
accompanied by exercises which should be done regularly
to maintain physical health.  These exercises are well
planned and do not require expensive equipment.

Throughout the book are scriptural phases which
authenticate God's hand in good nutrition.  The Bakers
say it beautifully in their own introduction--"The book
spells out the directions for maintaining or regaining
health.  They are simple.  They are direct.  Since they
come from our Creator, we can trust and follow them to
the letter and know that we will triumph."

This book is "must" reading and should be found in
every home in America.  I am proud to be part of the
monumental work.

Dr. Harold W. Manner, Ph.D.

# AFTERTHOUGHT

Every day more people are realizing that they must eat right to maintain health and conquer disease. They truly want to get off junk foods and onto an all-natural diet to bring this about, but they don't know where or how to start.

Before the time of Christ, the Roman Emperor, Tiberius, a great philosopher, said, "If anyone consult a doctor after the age of 30, he is a fool, since by that time everyone should know how to regulate his life properly."

In Hippocrates' time nutrition was held to be a major part of medical treatment and care. More recently Professor Arnold Ehret, an outstanding research scientist, therapist and writer whose works have been republished, considered nutrition extremely important in the care and recovery of his patients. The Father of American medicine, Sir William Osler, also believed strongly in sound nutritional principles.

Today, however, doctors aren't trained or encouraged to be much concerned about what a patient eats. Only a very few medical universities offer a course in nutrition and most of these are woefully inadequate.

In my lecturing to large audiences or small groups, in classes and consultations, I see a great need for help in breaking old eating habits and setting up new ones. Change rarely comes easy. I've received hundreds of letters from people who have read our UNCOOK BOOK. They are inspired by the raw food adventure, but many seek more specific guidance in changing from a health-suppressing diet to a health-giving one. I decided to meet that need.

THE UN-DIET BOOK is the result...a happy, how-to book with a program which leads step-by-step from a conventional diet to an all-natural one in seven easy phases. It encompasses the nutritional, spiritual and physical needs of The Complete Person.